The Physician's Role in Home Health Care

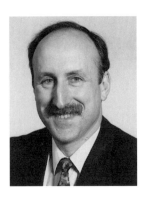 **Peter Avery Boling** is an Associate Professor of Internal Medicine at Virginia Commonwealth University, Medical College of Virginia, located in Richmond, Virginia. Years of home care experience and several thousand house calls fostered his interests in home care education, research, and policy development. He has conducted and published statewide and national surveys on physician home care practice and education, along with a variety of other scholarly writings. He has been a consultant to the American Medical Association, the Department of Veteran's Affairs, the National Association for Home Care, and several national home care companies. He is a technical expert on two current national studies of home care quality sponsored by the Health Care Financial Administration. November 1996 also marked the start of a 2-year term as President of the American Academy of Home Care Physicians. At home in Richmond, Dr. Boling maintains an active clinical practice that fills 60% of his time, including primary care office work, hospital rounds, nursing home care, and house calls. When he's not working, he enjoys the out-of-doors and the company of his wife Sue and their cat.

The Physician's Role in Home Health Care

Peter A. Boling, MD

Springer Publishing Company

Springer Publishing Company, Inc.
536 Broadway
New York, NY 10012–3955

Cover design by Margaret Dunin
Acquisitions Editor: Bill Tucker
Production Editor: Pamela Lankas

97 98 99 00 01 / 5 4 3 2 1

---

library of Congress Cataloging-in-Publication Data

Boling, Peter.
    The physician's role in home health care / Peter Boling.
      p.   cm.
    Includes bibliographical references and index.
    ISBN 0-8261-9700-0
    1. Home care services—United States. 2. Medicine—Practice—United States.
I. Title.
    [DNLM: 1. Home Care Services—United States. 2. Physician's Role.
WY 115 B689p 1997]
RA645.35.B65 1997
362.1'4'0973—dc21
DNLM/DLC
for Library of Congress   97-13704
                                               CIP

Printed in the United States of America

Contents

8 Home Health Care Delivery System Strategies
and Information Management   158

In Organized Systems How Does One Deliver Medical Care to
Functionally Impaired Community Dwellers? • On Lok and the
PACE Demonstration • The SHMO Experience • Other Managed
Care Systems • Life Care Communities • Rochester, New York:
Community-level Approaches • Home Hospitals • A Potpourri •
International Brethren • Creating a Viable System that Includes
Medical Home Care • Insurance Reform, System Reform, and
Vulnerable Populations • Information Management in Systems

Part III   Home Health Care in Our Society

9 Present and Projected Demands for Home Health Care   193

Who Will Need Home Health Care? • A Look at Some Basic
Demographics • Can We Forestall Frailty and Dependency by
Better Care? • Home Care for Those Who Are *Not* Chronically
Homebound • Defining Homebound • Population-Based
Studies of Dependency and Home Care Need • Closing Thoughts

10 Meeting the Demand for Home Health Care Services
in a Complex and Changing World   214

Determining the Number of Medical Home Health Care Providers
Needed • How Many Medical Providers Are Needed by the
Homebound? • Determining Provider House Call Capacity and
Caseload • Totaling up the Provider Picture • Selected Trouble
Spots: Underserved Areas and Missing Helpers • Possible Future
Effects on Supply and Demand • The "Frayed Edge": Moral and
Ethical Considerations in a Time of Shortage • Preparing to Face
Ethical Issues in Home Care • The Impact of Moral, Ethical, and
Social Concerns on Home Care Physicians

11 Education for Home Health Care   245

Neglect of Home Care Education • Creating and Using Oppor-
tunities for Home Care Education • What Should Be the Goals
of Home Health Care Education? • Current Undergraduate
(Medical Student) Home Care Education • Current Home Care
Education for Residents and Geriatric Fellows • Examples of
Residency Home Care Programs • Survey Data on Residency
Home Care Training • Personal Observations on Preparing
Young Physicians for Home Care • Home Care Education for

Foreword

The past decade has brought a dramatic change in the delivery of health care in America over the past decade. The needs of our aging population have generated innovative community-based options for long-term care. The Medicare prospective payment system in 1983, and more recently, the cost-containment pressures of managed care, have emptied our hospitals, shifting complex acute care to the outpatient and community setting. Sophisticated medical technology and professional services are now available in the home, allowing management of diseases previously cared for only in institutional settings. Almost as remarkable as these changes themselves is the noticeable lack of physician leadership and involvement in this transformation of health care back to the home.

Why aren't physicians at the center of this important transition in health care? Fifty years ago most physicians made home visits, and for many home care made up a substantial portion of their professional activity. The development of medical technology and the institutionalization of health care through the 1950s, 1960s, and 1970s has dramatically changed the practice and education of physicians. During those years home visits became obsolete and were considered less than community standard or "horse and buggy" medicine. Nonetheless, most of today's physicians regard home care as a useful and valuable service for their patients. Why then the disconnect? Why aren't physicians more involved in home care? Very few of the most recently trained generation of physicians have had any education or role modeling in home care. They are uncomfortable with their role in a home care practice and unfamiliar with general services available in the home. These barriers are further compounded by the financial disincentives associated with inadequate compensation for home care compared to other areas of physician work.

The phenomenal growth of home care shows every evidence of continuing well into the 21st century. With the acute management of medical problems in the home and the growing demands of long-term care, the need for active physician involvement is critical. For as long as there have been healers, the sick have been cared for in the home. Our present-day patients, especially the elderly, seem to again be expressing that preference. Physicians must become reacquainted with the traditions and values of healing in the home. That is why this book is so important and useful. It serves as a bridge and road map both back to the art of traditional home care and forward to the science and technology of modern home care. In many ways modern home care in our complex and regulated health systems is quite different from that practiced by our colleagues 50 years ago. Yet, Dr. Boling poignantly demonstrates how, in some of the most important ways, it hasn't changed at all. He is uniquely suited to author this volume as he combines the perspective of a clinician actively practicing home care and an academician who does research and teaching in home care, he is a leader in the American Academy of Home Care Physicians, and is a consultant to the home care industry and health policymakers. This is a welcome and timely book that will help physicians reestablish the art and science of home care.

JOSEPH KEENAN, MD

Acknowledgments

In preparing this manuscript I have been fortunate to have the advice and counsel of many colleagues. I would particularly mention Joseph Keenan, who read and critiqued an entire early draft; Sheldon Retchin, my mentor in health services research; and Joanne Schwartzberg, who taught me about regulations, policy, and politics. Later, Harry Wagner helped reorganize the book, and Mrs. Anne Brooks made the final revisions possible. During the past 2 years the support of my clinical colleagues during my periodic absences has also been invaluable. Finally, I must thank my wife and companion, Sue, for her patience, love, and encouragement. We put aside wilderness adventures and other personal goals to allow me the time I needed to write.

PART *I*

Home Health Care Physicians and What They Do

CHAPTER 1

Introduction

There are several excellent works on home care,[1-3] some of which describe physician practice.[4-8] Is another needed? To answer this, let me present the specific purposes for which this book was written. Although practice-based, it is *not* primarily a book to inform physicians about the details of home care practice. Other writers have described the clinical aspects of house calls and have extensively analyzed other home health services as a way of delivering care. These subjects are covered as background. Moreover, this is *not* a book about physician compensation, though I will write about incentives and financing. Physicians unfortunately have a reputation for affluence and self-interest that has hindered recent attempts at restoring them as members of the home care team.

Rather, this book is an attempt to better define the physician's role in home care. The role includes both house calls and work as a responsible member of an interdisciplinary team. I will try to make clear the connections between clinical home care experience, population demographics, and health services research while examining service provision, efficacy, and cost-effectiveness.

PHYSICIANS AND HOME HEALTH CARE

Physicians in the United States have become relatively invisible silent partners in home care. Although physicians are recognized as critical sources of referrals and medical support by the home health care industry, home care has received insufficient attention in medical education, research, and health policy. The physician's role has lost definition, lost value, and become misunderstood. However, the world is changing rapidly and home care needs more active physician involvement.[9]

Home care has many dimensions, ranging from chronic disease to acute illness, from bed baths to technologically complex therapy, from untrained caregivers to specialized professionals, from public housing to private mansions, and from urban settings to rural areas. At the turn of the 20th century physicians rode horses to the homes of patients with acute problems, delivered babies, treated epidemic infections and traumatic injuries, and helped with terminal care. Midcentury home care became a means for chronic care and postacute care, organized through public health departments and through hospitals seeking alternatives to prolonged inpatient care. Patient transportation improved. Mainstream medical practice became dominated by new technologies and facility-based therapies. The physician's role in home care gradually atrophied.

Now our society is aging, our concept of health care is changing, and home care is exploding. Chronic home care increases in company with the prevalence of frailty in the elderly, and acute, technologically advanced home care is an alternative to prohibitively costly hospital stays. Home care's tremendous growth requires physicians' active, informed participation. The aim of this book is to contribute to the future of the newly reemergent home care physician.

Take my case as an example. When I was a primary care internal medicine resident at the Medical College of Virginia, I signed many home health care orders, but like most residents, I had no grasp of what the orders meant, and I received no direct guidance. My real involvement with home care began in 1984, when I joined the faculty and was asked to start a house call program.

After 2 years of visiting patients in a variety of dwellings, making 15 or 20 house calls per week in the afternoons (after morning clinic sessions), and working to maintain continuity of care when these patients were hospitalized, I was exhausted. There was a huge community of patients, family members, and other home care professionals hungry for my help. Another world, characterized by poor reimbursement, provider shortages, and Machiavellian regulatory webs, had also become painfully familiar. There was a constant tension among obligations to my office practice, hospital, students, and academic colleagues, a tension familiar to physicians with multiple professional responsibilities.

Fortunately, an enlightened institution has made possible since 1987 the subsidized operation of an interdisciplinary home care team. The program was designed after programs built by pioneers in a field to which I was a newcomer. The team physicians, nurse practitioners, other helpers, and students have now made 18,000 house calls to over 750 homes.

During these 10 years of clinical work, I carefully studied home care and care delivery systems with the critical eye of an academic physician. Information from many sources and discussions of home health care with leaders in health services research, government, industry, and professional organizations form the underpinning of this book. These years have also seen the birth of the American Academy of Home Care Physicians, marking a new era for home care physicians.

THE SCOPE OF HOME HEALTH CARE

Discussions of home care, care management, or case management often begin with definitions. Home care certainly includes a heterogeneous variety of subsets, of which the roughly 2–3 million annual physician house calls and the related $100 million in expenses form only a tiny part.

Often distinguished from house calls by a different title, home health care typically denotes skilled professional-provider services delivered with physician oversight, including visits by nurses (47%), by therapists—physical (9%), occupational (1%), and speech (1%)—by social workers (less than 1%), and by others employed by home health agencies.[10] According to the Health Care Financing Administration (HCFA), this largest part of home care involved 228 million Medicare visits in 1995, increased from 127 million in 1992. The HCFA also reported that Medicare home health visits in 1994 cost $9.7 billion, with $7 billion more spent on Medicaid home care services.[11]

Basic supportive services provided by personal care aides or companions, high-tech services (e.g., infusion therapy, dialysis, or ventilator care), transportation, housing, and home medical equipment are other elements of broad-spectrum home health care. High-tech services are among the fastest-growing market sectors. In 1993 infusion therapy (62%), dialysis (29%), and respiratory therapy, including ventilator care (9%), generated $5.8 billion.[12]

Finally, there is the too often forgotten "informal" caregiver who does most of the work in home care.[13] Eighty percent of caregivers to the frail elderly provide unpaid assistance of some sort 7 days a week, averaging 4 hours per day.

Extrapolating from the 1987 National Medical Expenditure Survey, the aggregate cost of home care, not including the in-kind contributions of informal caregivers, housing, or transportation, was estimated to lie between $21 billion and $26 billion in 1993, or nearly 3% of all health care expenditures. Home care is big business.

HOW HOME HEALTH CARE ISSUES ARE TREATED IN THIS BOOK

Part I, "Home Health Care Physicians and What They Do," covers the role of physicians in home health care. These chapters discuss the physician's strengths and critical functions as a member of the home care team. They also discuss various other issues such as the following: How much of home care should be organized around a social model, as opposed to a medical model? Do homebound patients need doctors? Which home-bound patients need doctors? What should doctors do for homebound patients? How often and under what circumstances should doctors make house calls? How should doctors best interact with other home health professionals? Is home care a primary care activity, or do we need a cadre of "home care specialists"? How do physicians relate to nonmedical caregivers?

Part II, "Effectiveness, Organization and Management of Home Health Care," comprises three chapters dealing with the problems of systematizing home health care. Like "home care" the term "case management" has been used in many ways. Chapter 7, for instance, treats the ongoing process of patient evaluation, care planning, and patient reevaluation. Sometimes case management has a fiscal flavor, relating to the prudent use of resources; at other times a more clinical process is meant. Some prefer the term "care management," which sounds less impersonal and is preferred by patients or clients who do not like to be "cases" or have their lives "managed." These concerns aside, illnesses, treatments, and health care systems are so complex and costly that someone with exper-tise must be responsible for organizing the care to be provided to patients at home. With cost constraints becoming a focus and managed care expanding, physicians face an inevitable tension between practice goals and resource limitations. Weighing costs and patient needs to create cost-conscious or cost-effective treatment plans has become part of the physician's job.

Part III, "Home Health Care in Our Society," contains five chapters dealing with the various problems and opportunities home health care presents to the medical profession and to society in general. These chapters deal with such problems as the growing demand for home health care, the resources available to meet that demand, and the ethics of providing care in a time of shortage. Particularly interesting here is the issue of educating physicians about home health care. Medical education has advanced dramatically. Since the revolution of science in medicine, medical professionals now learn about subcellular mechanisms of disease, analysis of genes themselves, and therapies based on sophisticated molecular biology. Practitioners face an avalanche of information. In some ways it is not suprising that home care has seen less recent emphasis. The social ramifications of illness, particularly chronic illness, the complex interaction between home support and health, the availability of community resources, and the intricate payment mechanisms related to these services are areas in which most physicians are poorly versed. Can we expect physicians to know biology and psychology, yet also assimilate the extensive knowledge base specific to home care? Chapter 11 will address these concerns. Also discussed in Part III are the question of compensation for health care physicians and some thoughts on the future. I concentrate there on the needs of the next generation, those who will be frail in the year 2020, whose future physicians are now in school.

I hope that recommendations derived from this study of the physician's role in home care will find favor with colleagues and with those who make health policy. The home care needs of our society are rapidly increasing, demanding a robust structure of professional medical support in an integrated team model, including well-qualified home care physicians.

Because this exploration of the home care physician's role is rooted in clinical experience, I will start with an anecdote. A healthy, independent 90-year-old woman who was an office patient of mine for many years developed anaplastic thyroid cancer. This diagnosis followed on the heels of a hip fracture that left her nearly nonambulatory and forced her to move in with family. The cancer was growing rapidly, causing pain and trouble swallowing. Therapy for this aggressive cancer has little effect, so she was terminally ill. I spoke on the phone with the family about compassionate care at home. They asked me to visit, saying this would be very important for my patient, who counted heavily on her physician's advice. They lived in a rural area far from my office. I agreed to make one visit but told them I couldn't regularly travel this distance.

One hot August afternoon I drove 32 miles to a modest country home, accompanied by a fourth-year medical student. Two of my patient's children, senior citizens themselves, were there. Three others arrived within a few minutes, gathering behind us at the bedside. My patient, now nearly bedfast, was lying on her side. When I sat down, she reached out and spoke in a whisper, all that remained of her voice because the cancer was pressing on her windpipe. "Doctor, please help me. I'm suffering."

It was a moment one remembers and a time to teach without talking. The patient agreed to let her family make decisions about her care as long as I would treat her pain. I spent the next half hour teaching the family about pain control, about what to expect as she worsened, and about home care resources. We created a living will. She couldn't swallow pills, so I called local pharmacies to find one that stocked narcotic elixirs. As we were leaving, one daughter opened her checkbook and asked how much I wanted for my time, saying that the patient would ask if I was paid. I said I would bill Medicare, which is our office policy.

While we drove back to Richmond, the student and I talked. The value of this visit to the patient, to the family, and to me as a physician was obvious. We reviewed cancer pain management and community resources. Then we discussed the physician's role in home care and as a coordinator of care. The cold realities of efficiency, practice management, and financing contrasted sharply with the quality of our previous conversation. The student had earlier watched me hurry through clinic, hospital rounds, and administrative work. We had stopped to hospitalize a demented patient who unexpectedly appeared in the office just before we left, newly unable to walk. The student saw how it might be difficult to incorporate home care in a busy practice. Yet he couldn't reconcile his experience in this country home with a system that does not encourage physician involvement in home care. The challenge to the reader of this book is try to understand why we so badly need more physicians participating in home care, the form that this participation may take in an evolving health care system, and the changes in education and rewards that will be required.

REFERENCES

1. Spiegel AD. *Home Health Care.* 2nd ed. Owings Mills, MD: National Health Publishing; 1987.

2. Kane RA, Kane RL. *Long Term Care: Principles, Programs, and Policies.* New York: Springer Publishing Co; 1987: chaps 6, 7, 10.

3. Rowland D, Lyons B, ed. *Financing Home Care: Improving Protection for Disabled Elderly People.* Baltimore: Johns Hopkins University Press; 1991.

4. Hankwitz PE. Role of the physician in home care. *Physical Medicine and Rehabilitation* 1988; 2:289–305.

5. Bernstein LH, Grieco AJ, Dete M. *Primary Care in the Home.* Philadelphia: JB Lippincott Co.; 1987.

6. Keenan JM, Hepburn KW. The Role of Physicians in Home Care. *Clinics in Geriatric Medicine* 1991; 7:665–676.

7. Rossman I. The geriatrician and the homebound patient. *J Am Geriatr Soc.* 1988; 36:348–354.

8. Burton JR. The house call: An important service for the frail elderly. *J Am Geriatr Soc.* 1985; 33:291–293.

9. Vladeck BC. The Medicare home health initiative. *JAMA* 1994; 271:1566.

10. Chapter 6: Home Health Agency Benefits. *Health Care Financing Review.* 1992 Annual Supplement:137; 1992.

11. National Association for Home Care. *Basic Statistics about Home Care 1995;* Halamandaris V, editor. Washington DC: 1996.

12. Stern EM, Tidd GS. Health care reform's effect on home care: Strategies for survival. *Medical Interface.* May 1994; 85–90.

13. Stone R, Cafferata GL, Sangl J. Caregivers of the Frail Elderly: A National Profile. *Gerontologist* 1987; 27:616–626.

Attributes and Practices of the Home Health Care Physician

N o single job description defines the home health care physician. Instead there are several related roles. Most physicians who do home care work are based in ambulatory practice or hospitals. They oversee the home care delivered by home health agencies, and they provide few house calls. My practice is atypical. Few physicians, like those at the Medical College of Virginia (MCV) Home Care Program, have clinical roles that center around geriatric home care, make many housecalls to deliver primary care, and have broad home care skills. Only 2% of 1,161 internists and family physicians reported over 100 annual house calls in a recent national survey. Two physicians reported over 250 house calls (400 and 750).[1]

Other home care physicians have specialized practices, dealing selectively with home infusion therapy, home rehabilitation, emergency home care, home dialysis, home respiratory care, high-risk obstetrics, nutritional support, subspecialized pediatric care, or other such services. Finally, physicians are increasingly being recruited as medical directors of home health agencies or as consultants to payers, providers, and health systems. These are among the many different, legitimate roles for physicians in home care.

WHAT ARE THE ATTRIBUTES OF A
HOME HEALTH CARE PHYSICIAN?

There are common attributes that are shared by all good home care physicians. I offer here a baker's dozen, which I believe characterize the theoretical, ideal home care physician.

1. *Knowledgeable about home health care treatments and third-party coverage* Examples of treatments include professional care by nursing or physical therapy and others; home medical equipment; high-tech care like intravenous therapy, ventilators, or electronic home monitoring; and social services. Third-party coverage is complex and varies by payer, yet the basics must be understood.

2. *Broadly knowledgeable about pertinent medical issues* Such issues often involve medical problems prevalent in the functionally impaired elderly. Because it is often hard to obtain specialist consultations for the homebound, home care physicians need a broad range of medical skills. The patients present many common problems, often in advanced and refractory stages. Geriatric issues like dementia and delirium, incontinence, nutritional support, gait problems and falls, failure to thrive, end-of-life decisions, and bedsores (pressure ulcers) are common. Yet as comorbidity and heterogeneity increase with age, so one may encounter virtually any medical problem in the home. Nor is home care a geriatric activity. Pediatrics, psychiatry, obstetrics, neurology, and other fields all have important home care dimensions.

3. *Aware of caregiver issues* As patients become more dependent, caregivers increasingly become the focal point of care. Physicians must understand caregivers' issues at least as well as they understand patients' direct needs.

4. *Knowledgeable about pertinent medical ethics and legal issues* Common issues include decision making for the cognitively impaired, institutionalization, limiting life-sustaining therapies, and elder abuse.

5. *Knowledgeable about rehabilitation* Many home care patients are recovering from reversible conditions or have newly recognized conditions that may improve. The physician must first think of rehabilitation, then know how to initiate aggressive rehabilitative care, and finally recognize how to avoid inappropriate, futile efforts.

6. *Practical and flexible*   In home care one cannot solve every problem. The ability to rapidly determine sensible plans and solutions is vital. Closely related to practicality is flexibility, denoting willingness to adjust treatment plans, goals, and approaches as befits the situation. Environments that seem unacceptable to the physician may be adequate for the patient. Unorthodox caregiving strategies should often be accepted if they meet patients' basic needs and are not dangerous. Medication regimens may be adjusted to suit the home situation. Dietary indiscretions should sometimes be overlooked.

7. *Observant of the surroundings*   House calls offer a unique opportunity to examine the patient's environment for signs of correctable hazards and other clues that may improve care. Home care physicians need acute powers of observation.

8. *Compassionate*   There is much pain and suffering involved in chronic illness, for both patients and caregivers. Home care is no place for anyone lacking compassion.

9. *Mobile*   Physicians must periodically go into the home. They must have sufficient personal confidence, freedom in their schedule, familiarity with the roadways, and suitable transportation (usually a car) to facilitate house calls.

10. *Experienced*   Experience is important in any field. The independence required in home care work and the variety and complexity of medical, social, and ethical problems encountered make experience particularly valuable. Consider an analogy to cardiac surgery. There are obvious differences in the consequences of mistakes, yet experienced home care physicians deftly cut through tangled knots of problems in difficult home situations where those less experienced stumble and err.

11. *Effective communicator and educator*   Home care involves much explaining. It is replete with circumstances where the benefits of therapy are limited or where the benefit from treating one condition is counter balanced by possible ill-effects on other aspects of health. Caregivers and patients may differ about the best approach, and they raise many questions about medical issues. Physicians must be able to communicate with people in terms and language they can understand. This is harder than it sounds, and the difficulty is doubled by cultural or linguistic differences.

12. *Available*   This word is meant to suggest freedom to make house calls, plus being accessible by phone, Fax, pager, or other methods when needed by patients, caregivers, and other professionals. Covering physicians should also be available.

13. *Team player* Geriatricians emphasize interdisciplinary teams for good reasons. In addition to help from informal caregivers, homebound patients often need integrated care from several disciplines. Respect for team members and commitment to resolving the inevitable conflicts and process problems that arise are vital.

Few of these characteristics are unique to home care. Compassion, broad-based knowledge, experience, availability, commitment as a team player, and understanding of the relevant ethical framework are desirable in any physician. They are particularly important in primary care. Certain attributes, however, are specific to home care. Some are obvious, such as mobility, knowledge of home care services, and home care experience. With others, it is a matter of emphasis. For example, knowledge of geriatrics is used daily in most adult primary care practices, but greater geriatric sophistication may be required in home care, which is often dominated by frail older patients. Likewise, interdisciplinary teams in the office or hospital differ from home care, where team members are physically dispersed and the team involves more people who do not know each other well.

THE CLINICAL KNOWLEDGE AND TRAINING OF A HOME HEALTH CARE PHYSICIAN

Obviously, effective home care physicians must know community resources, the capabilities and limitations of interdisciplinary home care teams, physician contributions to team efforts, how to be a team player, and pertinent regulations for services by home health agencies and home medical equipment providers. Fully acquiring this knowledge base takes years.

Medical knowledge and skills specific to home care are also needed. Providers can use knowledge developed for nursing homes, hospitals, and ambulatory settings, but home care requires modifications. Though the patients are similar, physician knowledge and skills for nursing homes are not entirely interchangeable with those used in home care.

One example is pressure ulcer care. The wounds are similar in character and causation, but therapy at home may require different choices. Who will change the dressing at home and how often? Whirlpool baths are difficult. On the other hand, some patients are repositioned more reliably at home if they have "one-on-one" care from family members.

Then consider dementia. Like physicians directing nursing home Alzheimer's disease units, home care physicians encounter wandering, reversal of sleep-wake cycles, angry outbursts, and socialization issues. Nursing home physicians face problems that are rare in home care, such as having many demented people in one place, inappropriate sexual behavior, and liability. On the other hand, nursing homes have more resources. There are electronic door alarms, and trained caregivers are always present. The environment is relatively controlled, uniform, and unchanging. Compared with home care, nursing home physicians less often debate the safety of patients remaining at home or medicating patients so that caregivers can rest. The challenges are different.

Adult homes, or board-and-care facilities, fall somewhere between nursing homes and home care. Adult homes are like nursing homes in that they are group dwellings with a staff always on site, but they are far less regulated and less intensive in their staffing and services. Some commonly used physician home care capabilities are discussed below.

Comprehensive Functional Assessment

Evaluating daily function is central to home care. This is an important practice for physicians working in offices or hospitals who need to recognize basic home care needs and will do so most often by noting that the patient's ability to function is impaired. The need for more extensive functional assessment is typical for homebound patients of all ages because the concurrent presence of several comorbid illnesses and diminished functional status are universal. With aging, illness presentation often becomes less typical, and functional status becomes even more important both to detecting problems and to marking progress.

Medication Management

Most physicians are familiar with medication noncompliance and its relation to adverse events. One study found that 11% of elderly patient hospitalizations involved medication compliance.[2] Conversely, I have seen many cases where patients avoided serious problems by stopping prescribed medications; these events are hard to count. In home care, noncompliance is a major concern. Physicians must know about pillboxes, which pharmacies deliver, and know about the many factors that affect know compliance. Pharmacists can help with delivery and pillboxes and also can function as consultants,[3] either by phone or as members of home care teams. This has been recognized since the 1970s. Medications may have to be changed to accommodate the needs of the family, to simplify care. Compared with the hospital, the medication regimen is usually less sacrosanct when seen in action at home.

Nutrition

Recognizing undernutrition is important, because patients with poor nutrition do poorly,[4] and poor nutrition can be subtle. Once undernutrition is identified, physicians must know how to plan affordable calorie supplements and, if necessary, nasogastric or gastrostomy feedings, choosing among numerous commercial formulas. It is sometimes sufficient to review the diet and teach the family to puree food, estimate calories, or prepare appealing meals.

Problems with feeding tubes are also common. What does one do when the gastrostomy leaks near the opening or greenish drainage and traces of blood appear at the hole? What should happen if the tube cracks? How long do tubes last before they need replacement, and what type of tube is best? Rigid feeding schedules established according to hospital routines are not necessary at home. I am always amused by how much institutional tube feeding routines differ from the nutritional patterns of people's daily lives. With proper attention to preventing aspiration and hunger, feeding schedules can be arranged around caregiver needs. Drickamer and Cooney give useful advice about enteral feeding.[5]

Incontinence and Urinary Catheter Management

Often, incontinent women who are relatively mobile can be kept dry. This is less true in home care. After trying a voiding schedule, a commode chair, and medication changes, one is often left with persistent incontinence. Ordering disposable diapers and Chux simply requires paperwork. However, the decision to insert a bladder catheter is more difficult, involving the juxtaposed risks of infection and nonhealing wounds. Subsequently, the physician will be asked about the frequency of catheter changes, choice of catheter type, use of bladder irrigations, problems with urine leaking around the catheter, how to handle cloudy sediment, and whether the recent downturn in functional status represents an infection in a bladder that is chronically overgrown with bacteria. Nurses often call to ask about antibiotic therapy.

Wound Care

Most postoperative wounds heal quickly at home, but pressure ulcers, venous stasis, and arterial ulcers can persist for years. A baffling array of wound care products are available. Sophisticated, expensive beds with low-air-loss and air-fluidized mattresses are part of the home care armamentarium, and physicians must learn when and how they should be used.[6,7] Many physicians count on nurses to guide wound care, yet knowledge of basic principles in wound healing is necessary for effective partnership.

Psychiatric Problems

Psychiatrically impaired homebound patients became numerous with the sharp reduction of institutional psychiatric care in the 1970s. These patients present a unique set of challenges,[8] often better met by mobile, community-based teams.[9,10] Home care is coming to the forefront as a means of preventing acute crises and hospitalizations for chronically ill psychiatric patients.[11]

The homebound have a high prevalence of dementia, depression, anxiety, substance abuse, psychosis, and agoraphobia, affecting both geriatric[12] and younger patients. Some home health agencies provide psychiatric home care, covered by Medicare and Medicaid under selected circumstances, and some managed care systems are venturing into psychiatric home care. However, most homebound patients have trouble accessing good longitudinal psychiatric care, so nonpsychiatric home care physicians often manage these complex problems. Knowing psychopharmacology is important, as is knowing when not to prescribe.

Respiratory Care, Tracheostomy Care, Ventilator Care

The simpler part of home respiratory care is prescribing oxygen for patients with chronic lung and heart disease. One must know the rationale and regulations governing eligibility, but several questions remain. How reliable is home oximetry?[13] Who needs portable oxygen and who can manage with a concentrator alone? When should oxygen be moisturized? Which patients should get transtracheal oxygen? Respiratory therapists can be of great help, but once again physicians need some basic knowledge. Another common therapy is nebulizer treatment for bronchodilation, secretion control, or preventing pneumocystis pneumonia in AIDS patients. These are straightforward once you know the ropes. Tracheostomy care can also be straightforward but can quickly become complicated or even fatal. Ventilator care is similar: When patients are stable it is easy; but when troubles come, situations can suddenly be very difficult. Even with stable patients, home ventilator care has broad psychological, ethical, and fiscal dimensions.[14]

Pediatric Home Care

A few children have severe chronic illnesses. Pediatric home respiratory, tracheostomy, and ventilator care are a new frontier.[15] Babies who were premature sometimes have respiratory problems like bronchopulmonary dysplasia. Patients with advanced cystic fibrosis also present home respiratory therapy challenges. Other children depend on sophisticated nutritional support, including long-term parenteral (intravenous) feeding, following catastrophic events such as newborn necrotizing enterocolitis.

Pregnancy

Some women with routine pregnancies prefer home delivery, which is safe in good hands.[16] Threatened or otherwise complicated pregnancies are a new area for home care, and the related technology is still being studied.[17] Many women now receive tocolytic therapy at home (low-dose infusion of terbutaline to stop premature labor) or home management for hypertension, preeclampsia, and hyperemesis gravidarum (protracted vomiting that requires intravenous hydration). These patients require a specialized approach.

Spinal Cord and Brain Injury

There is a fairly large group of homebound people who have suffered spinal cord and central nervous system injury. They are often younger than other home care patients, and they require specialized management for muscle spasticity, bowel and bladder care, blood pressure instability, seizures, and related complications.

AIDS and Related Problems

AIDS patients in home care form a special group. When homebound, AIDS patients are often in a brief, terminal phase of life, receiving comfort care. Earlier in the illness, AIDS patients have various home care needs, including infusion therapy and nutritional support. Many receive toxic medications at home, like gancyclovir or amphotericin B, which require expertise. The late complications of AIDS include complex disorders unfamiliar to many physicians, such as progressive multifocal leukoencephalopathy (PML), AIDS wasting syndrome, refractory diarrhea, assorted unusual infections, lymphomas, and disseminated Kaposi's sarcoma. Finally, while the caregivers' and professional home care providers' risk of exposure to the AIDS virus is very low, the possibility is frightening, even to many experienced home care professionals, and remains a barrier to expanding AIDS home care. Exposure to strains of tuberculosis resistant to most antituberculosis drugs is another new and potentially serious risk.

Home Infusion

This domain crosses several of those mentioned above, requiring familiarity with intravenous access devices like peripherally inserted central catheters (PICC) or semipermanent central vein catheters (e.g., Hohn, Hickman, or Groshong) and knowing when home infusion is safe and appropriate. To some extent these problems distinguish home care from inpatient care, in which simpler temporary peripheral intravenous lines are the rule. The first request to authorize infusion of urokinase or hydrochloric acid to clear a central line at home exemplifies an order that may cause an inexperienced physician some anxiety.

Telephone Medicine

Though it is daily fare in office practice, telephone work has special importance for home care. Home care physicians daily make "triage" decisions that involve serious problems and control expensive resources: home health agency visits, house calls, home medical equipment use, ambulance transport, and emergency room care. Thus, they must be adept at discerning the nature and severity of problems on the telephone. Interestingly, formal teaching of telephone medical skills is only now entering residency curricula for office practice.

Knowing When to Stop

Despite experts who support cardiopulmonary resuscitation (CPR) for healthier older patients, there is overwhelming evidence that chronically ill patients with poor baseline functional status, often elderly, have dismal results from CPR. This is true at home, in the hospital, and in long-term residential care settings.[18] The likelihood of restoring both basic life functions *and* baseline functional status is often 1% or less, and half of those who survive may be severely neurologically impaired, a fate many consider worse than death. Thus, an important part of home care is knowing when to be less aggressive and communicating that understanding to families who may fear the nearness of death. This takes practice, familiarity with the facts, and interpersonal skills. Similar issues arise with decisions about other aggressive therapies, like major surgery or dialysis.

Legal and Ethical Dimensions

Because much of home care involves the end of life and the limits of medical capability to reverse illness, issues like do-not-resuscitate (DNR) orders, living wills, and even passive or active euthanasia are often raised. When, if ever, can you stop tube feedings or simply allow someone to die at home of dehydration without inserting a tube? When is it ethical to withhold antibiotics in the face of serious infection? Is it legal? What local laws govern the implementation of prehospital DNR orders? In Virginia a recent law restricted DNR orders to persons with a "terminal" diagnosis or a persistent vegetative state. Someone with end-stage emphysema and the possibility of living another 10 years could not legally declare himself DNR, during ambulance transport, nor could a spouse legally stop the ambulance team from resuscitation, even with a living will. Two years later, this potentially unconstitutional law was amended.

Then, what about forcibly removing patients from home because they are "dangerous" to themselves or to others? This gray zone complicates many discussions at MCV Home Care team meetings and is addressed further in chapter 11. When is there sufficient evidence of abuse or neglect for Adult Protective Service representatives to take action? When is a situation simply deplorable but not actionable?

Terminal Care

Care of the dying is a substantial part of home care practice; here ideal physician attributes include compassion, emphasis on caring and comfort rather than cure, understanding of the psychological dimensions of loss and grief, and skill at controlling pain.[19,20] Terminal care has been epitomized by dying cancer patients.[21] However, most terminal illness stems from other common problems like heart failure, emphysema, cirrhosis, kidney failure, and stroke. One helpful service is simply to prepare the family for the details at the death scene itself and discussing whom they should call; these are details that often create needless anxiety.

Rehabilitation

Physiatry is another area where home care generalists must be capable, without necessarily being experts. It is vital to recognize patients with potential for restoring function or with high-risk conditions, like recent immobilization of joints, early contractures, and deconditioning after serious illness. Prompt action can prevent grave consequences. For example, I am treating a woman who was reportedly ambulatory, though demented, 3 months earlier when she fell. Three months before she moved to Richmond she had become bedfast, with deep decubitus ulcers over both greater trochanters and the sacrum. There was no clear evidence of a paralyzing neurological or orthopedic injury, yet her immobility and her wounds had become severe and intractable. It required 2 years for her skin to heal. Focus on functional status and the time course of events is crucial.[22]

Home Medical Equipment

Jay Portnow is a leader in home rehabilitation, and his writings may define the standard for physician work with home medical equipment.[23] His series of recent articles in the *American Academy of Home Care Physicians Newsletter* (1992–1994) provide a useful review of many medical equipment options. This work is now extended in a separate newsletter called *Durable Medical Equipment Review.*

Home medical equipment prescribing has become a larger aspect of physicians' home care work because of the 1990 OBRA law, mandating that physicians complete certificates of medical necessity (CMNs) for durable medical equipment and the new durable medical equipment regional carrier (DMERC) program, implemented to standardize coverage policy and ensure more appropriate use of home medical equipment. Eleven CMN forms, including one for oxygen, now cover all home medical equipment, forms that physicians need to understand.[24]

The DMERC process requires patient-specific information from physicians, in addition to their signatures on the CMNs. Many physicians are poorly informed about home medical equipment after years of relying on vendors and other home health professionals. Since 1994 the DMERCs, assisted by the Health Industry Distributors Association, the National Association of Medical Equipment Suppliers, the American Academy of Home Care Physicians, and others have been revising the process of certification to maintain control over utilization while simplifying the administrative work.

Physicians prescribing home medical equipment should know about basic wheelchairs, commodes, and hospital beds and what conditions require their use. Physicians should also resist inappropriate requests from those few vendors who continue to abuse the system. To assist physicians, an information sheet about each piece of equipment is being developed that may accompany some CMNs. However, it is clear that physiatrists, home physical and occupational therapists, and responsible home medical equipment vendors will remain the experts and principal advisors when prescribing more sophisticated devices.

HOME CARE: GENERALIST FIELD OR SPECIALTY FIELD?

Is home care practice a generalist or specialist activity? This question recalls the debate now embroiling geriatrics,[25] obstetrics/gynecology, and other disciplines. The answer is simple, but it does not resolve the debate. Home care is a field for *both* specialists and generalists.

Giving home care to complex frail patients requires specialized knowledge and experience. When I am involved in such cases, I bring a carefully built knowledge base specific to home care and a capability to efficiently solve home care problems that many excellent generalists lack. The concept of relative specialization in home care is valid even when using basic home care technology and simple medical therapy. By contrast, my knowledge of ambulatory AIDS care is less advanced; most AIDS patients in our system attend a clinic designed for AIDS care.

At the same time, home care practice epitomizes generalism and primary care, being, as it is, holistic, humanistic, observational, empirical, intuitive, community-oriented, continuous, and broad in clinical scope. It is a patient-centered activity, emphasizing empathy, understanding, and communication skills. Primary care physicians often handle complex secondary and tertiary problems, using approaches that differ from those of specialists. Home care patients also tend to have several active problems, making it difficult for a group of specialists to provide coordinated care if each specialty handles only one limited aspect of the case.

Consider IT, a woman in her 80s referred to me for geriatric primary care by a vascular surgeon who managed her lower extremity arterial insufficiency. IT was very weak and short-winded. My colleague was uncomfortable, thinking she might need hospitalization. The cardiologist who recently treated IT at a local hospital had reportedly told the family there was nothing more he could do for IT and that she should find a generalist.

The medical problem list was impressive. In addition to severe arterial disease, IT had end-stage emphysema requiring home oxygen, a severe hypertrophic cardiomyopathy, episodes of acute atrial tachycardia causing heart failure, leg swelling from several problems combined, urinary incontinence, osteoporosis, arthritis, and poor nutrition. Lab work showed some kidney failure. On exam, IT was thin, wasted, weak, and visibly short of breath from any activity. Her legs felt cool, were moderately swollen, and had numerous sores. She was, however, articulate and in full command of her thoughts. Her life was lived on a couch, from which she gingerly walked 5 feet to the adjacent bathroom.

In the emergency room where we first met, it took only a few minutes to see that IT was fairly stable, with severe chronic problems, none of which would benefit from hospital care. There had apparently been no satisfactory prior exploration of the expectations, desires, goals, and needs of the patient and family. It was clear that IT was resigned to the approaching end of life. She wanted to be supported and made comfortable. She wanted to stay at home on her couch, and she needed an advocate to help make that possible.

IT's precarious situation put her primary caregiver in a state of chronic anxiety, afraid that she would make a mistake and cause irreparable harm and unsure how to respond when IT's condition changed. The caregiver's natural response to apparent crises was to seek medical care, often at an emergency room. She needed someone to advise her when she faced difficulties. She had her own physical problems, limiting her ability to handle the increasing physical strain of IT's care. I made it clear to her during our first talk that the focus should be comfort, not cure. This was readily accepted as long as I would be available to help work through any issues that might arise. I must acknowledge parenthetically that in this regard I benefited from the previous attempts at medical miracles by the cardiologist at the other hospital. The patient and family were already convinced that medicine had no definitive answer for IT's problems.

Obviously, the knowledge and skills germane to such a case involve several domains. The first is competence with complex medical problems and related questions. IT had severe lung disease, heart disease with rhythm disturbances and pump failure, kidney problems, and advanced arterial disease, plus "geriatric" problems like osteoporosis, poor nutrition, functional incontinence, and deconditioning. She took several potent, potentially toxic medications for these problems.

The second involves understanding of caregiver needs and burdens and anticipating reactions to new problems. A letter that came from this grateful caregiver after IT died is reproduced in chapter 5. It clarifies the value of physician support to the caregiver. The third domain required knowledge of legal and ethical principles related to preferences for limiting care and skill in counseling families through terminal care. Finally, there was the need to know about community resources and how to arrange and coordinate home care. This patient was eligible for additional home care services.

Considered in this light, it is easy to understand why I felt like a specialist as I quickly discovered the needs and devised a plan for care at home. The exploration, discovery, and treatment felt almost surgical as the anatomy of a complex problem was dissected and the relief was immediately perceptible, without a single medical intervention. What I newly offered were some extra home care services and my continuing advice and support. Yet what I did was the home care physician's equivalent of initiating cardiopulmonary bypass, the first stage of a complicated operation.

On the other hand, much of my generalist orientation and training were vital, augmented by specialized knowledge and experience specific to home care, in this instance terminal care. Was I serving as a generalist or a specialist? The answer is, both. If forced to choose for political reasons, I would say that the primary care aspects of home care outweigh the specialist aspects in most cases.

SUBSPECIALTY AND HIGH-TECH HOME CARE

On behalf of my more technology-oriented home care colleagues, I note that some elements of home care, elements not used by IT, are very technical indeed, such as home infusion of chemotherapy or dobutamine, home ventilator care, or home dialysis. Often, these are best directed by subspecialized physicians: cardiologists may oversee home dobutamine infusion; nephrologists may direct home dialysis; oncologists may supervise home chemotherapy; infectious disease consultants may manage home infusion therapy programs; pulmonologists may oversee home ventilator care; and gastroenterologists may order home nutrition. Of course, subspecialists who successfully direct home care cannot do this with a hospital or office specialist's perspective. They must learn about home care, which is different. Nevertheless, involvement of subspecialists in home care has two particular values. First, many primary care physicians lack the interest or expertise to direct the more technical aspects of home care. Second, there are always some situations where even technically sophisticated primary care physicians need help.

There are, fortunately, developed oases of subspecialty home care. For example, in the early 1980s oncologist Khalid Mahmud developed CareVan, a home infusion service that later became MEDISYS. This was the vehicle for study of new approaches such as using intravenous heparin at home for anticoagulant therapy of deep vein thromboses.[26] Emphasizing quality and avoiding conflicts of interest and unethical behavior that enmired some competitors,[27] CareVan provided much valuable care.

Home infusion therapy has been championed by many strong voices. Poretz and colleagues at Fairfax Hospital have enormous experience, and provide excellent reviews,[28] as does Tice.[29] Starting in the 1970s, antibiotics for chronic infections were among the first home intravenous therapies, including treatment of children with osteomyelitis or cystic fibrosis. Other early explorations involved home transfusions; parenteral nutrition, which can improve quality of life,[30] and infusion of narcotics for pain management. The success of home infusion has driven an explosive market, and while noting the need to ensure appropriateness and provider quality, the Office of Technology Assessment (1992) endorsed wider use of home infusion, potentially including Medicare coverage.[31]

New technologies are expanding the range of home infusion therapy.[32] These include new medications, like low-molecular-weight heparin,[33,34] and techniques for opening occluded venous catheters.[35] In Great Britain, general practitioners are giving thrombolytic therapy at home for patients with suspected acute myocardial infarction and reporting a 50% reduction in mortality at 1 year.[36]

Home hemodialysis is another therapy used selectively since the mid 1960s, complementing continuous ambulatory peritoneal dialysis as home care options for patients who require dialysis and can manage complex procedures.

Home rehabilitation has advanced principally as a branch of home health agency care, but physicians like Jay Portnow have moved comprehensive rehabilitative care into the home. The founder of Wellmark, Dr. Portnow is an expert in effectively providing services at home that were considered the domain of inpatient rehabilitation units.

Pediatric home ventilator care and other advanced respiratory support systems have long interested Allen Goldberg.[37] In detailing the care provided to 18 ventilator-dependent children in the Northwestern University pediatric home ventilator program, Goldberg argues for active involvement of medical specialists in home care. Many experts, including those at the University of Pennsylvania[38] (21 cases) and Baylor[39] (54 cases) concur.

Emergency home care is developing through the efforts of innovators like Gresham Bayne, who directs Call Doctor, Inc. His company's vans contain X-ray, ECG, and lab equipment, plus a technician-driver and a physician, allowing immediate and complete evaluation and stabilization of seriously ill patients. Communicating by modem, these providers can be integrated into a complete delivery system, avoiding the need for many ambulance trips.

Home obstetrical and perinatal care now includes use of prolonged low-dose terbutaline infusion to prevent premature delivery.[40] And babies born with neonatal jaundice can have bilirubin light therapy at home, saving days of inpatient care and placing child and mother together at home with less artificial separation. Such new therapies are having typical growing pains.[41]

WHEN DO GENERALISTS DIRECT
SPECIALIZED HOME CARE?

Still, these exceptional specialty services constitute only a small fraction of home care and are not universally available. Most involve technical, often longitudinal therapy that is relatively well-reimbursed rather than generic or intermittent consults for diagnosis and care planning. Accordingly, until more physicians are involved in home care, including subspecialists, it will be up to home care generalists to solve complex, specialized problems for home care patients. Fortunately, while specialists are very helpful, generalists are often able to direct highly specialized home care. Home antibiotic therapy, narcotic infusions for pain control, ventilator care, and enteral nutrition are part of my own home care practice. I am grateful to have a strong group of subspecialists available for advice. They in turn seem glad that I will handle the many other inevitable complexities of long-term home care that would otherwise fall on their shoulders. We complement each other. I still wish they would make more consultative house calls.

Following is a case that shows what generalists can sometimes handle. BJ was a 62-year-old woman with emphysema. Mechanical ventilation started in the hospital, and she could not be weaned from the ventilator. She felt that she was not ready to die, so she had a tracheostomy and was prepared for home ventilator care, with help from her husband. She was referred to me for longitudinal care in 1986.

This poor African American couple lived in a dilapidated old house a mile from the hospital. She was tiny and so weak that she could barely stand up in the second-floor bedroom. Her nutrition had deteriorated, the loss of appetite perhaps aggravated by the belief that her husband was seeing other women in his first-floor apartment. Still, she wanted to live and was also determined to be free of the ventilator. Against my advice, she stopped ventilatory support and had the equipment company retrieve the machine. Soon she was in bad shape, yet she refused emergency room care. Her husband called, exhausted and desperate after providing manual ventilation with an Ambu bag for 36 consecutive hours. I saw her at home immediately. Her blood pressure was low, and she was drowsy from elevated levels of carbon dioxide in her blood. Her legs and feet, once bone-thin, were swollen to the waist from right heart failure induced by low blood oxygen levels.

BJ had been adamant about staying at home. Even in her delirium she resisted hospitalization, while maintaining that she was not ready to die. Her husband supported her desire to stay home. The ventilator was the only option, one she would now accept because the alternative was death. I warned them that we would run a serious risk of a poor outcome in trying to restart ventilatory support at home under these conditions, but they were determined. I drew blood, including an arterial blood gas, which I packed in ice cubes from the refrigerator. The lab results looked terrible: severe respiratory failure with advanced acidosis, kidney failure from low blood flow, and markedly abnormal potassium levels.

The equipment company reinstalled the ventilator, and blood gasses were taken every 4 hours for the first day, with daily measurements of other labs. Diuretics started to reduce the edema as the ventilator allowed her metabolic abnormalities to reverse. Soon she was stable: a medical home care success. Though sometimes miserable and depressed, at other times she was cheerful and content. She died quietly at home 3 years later.

I would also mention HL, our most difficult home ventilator patient, to show that although technical knowledge is needed in high tech cases, non-technical aspects often dominate the work. After a turbulent adolescence, HL suffered severe head trauma and a broken neck in an accident, leaving him quadriplegic and ventilator-dependent. Following lengthy rehabilitation, HL was moved to his parents' home along with his two young children; his wife had left him long before.

Taking 12-hour shifts, HL's parents gave care reminiscent of an intensive care unit. They were determined that he would not go to a nursing home. He required tracheal suctioning, tube feedings, suprapubic urinary catheter management, bowel care, bathing, blood pressure monitoring, and tilt table exercises for blood pressure instability related to the spinal cord damage. He had a chronic central venous catheter. The head trauma and loss of independence caused HL emotional, cognitive, and behavioral problems and made communication difficult. Yet he was alert and sometimes expressed himself very clearly.

The parents were dedicated, but they lacked medical background and needed frequent help to understand and solve the many problems their son presented. These included seizure-like episodes; ventilator and tracheostomy problems; expressions of angry, crazy feelings; sleeplessness; limited attempts to generate speech using mechanical devices; and infections, including a chronic bone infection that eventually required surgery and home intravenous antibiotics. There were many phone calls; each new observation might indicate a serious medical problem, though most did not, thus requiring skilled decision making. HL's parents were unrealistically hopeful that he would regain function, causing them anxiety when he had setbacks. As time passed and they tired, their need for progress intensified even as they increasingly recognized intransigence of HL's problems.

Moving HL was a major project. To leave home, he required "bagging" (manual ventilation), facilities for suctioning, and a portable ventilator. Ambulances and emergency rooms are equipped for such cases, but physicians' offices are not, so consultations were very difficult. Most problems were addressed at home by me with help from respiratory and speech therapists. After 4 years of home care, HL died during a tracheostomy tube change when the family was unable to insert a new airway. Thus, the hardest aspects of the case were not technical issues like the ventilator and the voice computer that HL refused to use. Rather, they were the neuropsychiatric disturbances and managing the family's needs, questions, and demands.

These high-tech cases involved a ventilator, a form of therapy with which I am reasonably comfortable after a strong intensive care unit experience during residency, though I am by no means a respiratory care expert. Other technology-intensive therapies, such as intravenous medication, gastrostomy feeding, and suprapubic catheter care are also familiar to me. Some procedures, like dialysis, would make me uncomfortable. Other primary care physicians might be less comfortable with the ventilator cases described above, depending on their training and experience. Each physician has strengths and limits. Each can learn new therapies if circumstance demands. I have learned much during my home care years.

THE COMPETING DEMANDS ON HOME CARE PHYSICIANS

This section describes the differing demands home care physicians face each day, identifying contributions physicians can make in home care and circumstances where active participation is important. Other writers have broached this subject,[42–45] yet after talking with many colleagues, health administrators, and payers, I find that most people simply do not understand the actual work of a home care physician.

Most physicians involved in home care have other professional responsibilities that far outweigh their home care work, a circumstance that makes a necessity of balancing priorities. This has been clearly voiced in many physician surveys. A recent national survey of internists and family physicians (1,161 responses) with active outpatient practices (10 or more office hours per week) regarding home care activities, found attitudes favoring house calls while also capturing the flavor of competing priorities.[1] See Table 2.1.

Continuing with a quantitative approach, general internists nationally reported an average work week with 56 hours of patient care.[46] This workload has been stable for years and compares closely with family physicians, general practitioners, surgeons, pediatricians, and most other

TABLE 2.1 Percentage Responding Agree or Strongly Agree

Physician attitude	Physicians who make house calls	Physicians who don't make house calls
Physician house calls are an important service for selected patients.	93	69
I am too busy with office or hospitalpractice to make house calls.	47	80
With readily available visiting registered nurses and nursing aides, most home visits by physicians are unnecessary.	48	70
Physicians should use home health agencies more.	85	84

From "A National Survey of the Home Visiting Practice & Attitudes of Family Physicians & Internists," by Keenan et al., 1992, *Archives of Internal Medicine, 152*, 2025–2032. Copyright © 1992, American Medical Association. Printed with permission.

disciplines. Direct patient care constitutes 89% of internists' reported work. This includes 27 hours of office practice, 15 hours of hospital work, and 7 hours for other direct patient care. Family physicians report 35 hours in the office and 7 hours in the hospital, reflecting traditional differences between the disciplines.

During a typical day, an office-based physician sees patients at 15- or 20-minute intervals, totaling 20 to 30 daily visits, or 112 (internist) to 146 (family physician) visits per week. Such practices might have 2,500 active cases under fee-for-service or 1,800 cases under managed care, which creates extra demands. Attendant on the office visits is much paper and telephone work. There are lab reports to review; correspondence with consultants to read or dictate, as well as phone calls from patients, families, and other professionals; disability and insurance forms to complete; and assorted other administrative tasks.

Then comes acute care. When patients become acutely ill, office-based physicians must respond. Fitting acute care into the day is difficult because it is time-consuming and unpredictable. Accordingly, physicians have plans for handling acute care. Sometimes, emergency department physicians and inpatient consultants manage all acute care. On the other end of a spectrum are primary care physicians who personally handle most emergent care. In many groups, physicians alternate outpatient work with days or weeks of acute care, taking turns "protecting" the office from disruptive effects imposed by acute problems. Then, "howdy rounds," or visiting patients in the hospital after office hours when one is not directing the care, may become the means of maintaining the doctor-patient relationship.

Many generalists also practice in long-term care facilities, an activity that is usually planned or scheduled, often seeing several patients under one roof. However, nursing home patients and their families present unexpected demands. Patients develop fevers or fall and require urgent in-person physician evaluation following initial telephone orders. The evaluations often occur after office hours.

Into this sea of crossing currents we introduce home care. Home care patients may be in the practice because of deteriorating health after years of office-based care, they may meet the physician for the first time in the hospital, or they may be referred specifically for physician home care. Regardless of their point of origin, home care patients bring their own set of needs. From the perspective of competing priorities, home care is like nursing home care, but there are critical differences. Unlike nursing homes, where patients can be checked frequently by nurses, most home care patients receive only sporadic professional observation. Physicians and unpaid caregivers have greater responsibility, and this may increase the urgency for definitive physician evaluation.

The 1990 national telephone survey explored urgent home care.[1] We asked: "If one of your established homebound patients calls you at your office with an acute complaint that's not an emergency, what would you ordinarily do or recommend?" Respondents were given time to answer. If needed, they were given choices. Table 2.2. shows how priorities and approaches differ when physicians are confronted with an acute home care problem.

WHERE HOME CARE PHYSICIANS' TIME IS SPENT

In this survey the average respondent was a 44-year-old male, working 63 hours per week with 55 hours of patient care. Half made house calls but

TABLE 2.2 Approach to the Acute but Nonemergent Home Care Patient

Option	Percentage selecting option
Send patient to ER by ambulance	16
Send patient to office by ambulance/van	20
Schedule nursing visit by home health agency	15
Schedule physician home visit	15
Send office nurse, nurse practitioner, or physician assistant to the home	3
Other (e.g., telephone management)	30

From "A National Survey of the Home Visiting Practice & Attitudes of Family Physicians & Internists," by Keenan et al., 1992, *Archives of Internal Medicine, 152*, 2025–2032. Copyright © 1992, American Medical Association. Reprinted with permission.

averaged only 9 per year while estimating that they followed 21 home-bound patients. "Homebound" was defined as "individuals who can leave home only with considerable or taxing effort or with the assistance of another individual or device." Even with a standard definition, it is hard to know if the phrase "homebound patient" would conjure the same image for a family physician in Kansas City or a general internist in Klamath Falls, Oregon, as it does for me in Richmond. Still, let's assume some similarity and borrow from other sources plus my experience, which suggest that a caseload of 150 medically ill homebound patients can constitute a full-time job for one physician (see chapters 9 and 10 for details). This presumes that patients receive physician attention comparable to what they would receive if they came to the office or lived in nursing homes. It would also make the reported average of 21 homebound patients a substantial part of one physician's work, perhaps 10% or more.

It may seem far-fetched that so few patients could consume so much time until you follow a home care physician's footsteps. This was done in a time–motion study during the Rochester Home Health Care Team randomized experiment.[47] The team managed seriously ill patients, a third of whom died, with an average census of 54. Also the team members—a physician, a nurse practitioner, and a social worker—had responsibilities

TABLE 2.3 Rochester Home Health Care Team (Percentage of Work Time)

Variable	Physician	Nurse practitioner	Social worker
Direct patient contact			
Home	22.7	28.0	23.2
Hospital	15.4	7.3	1.6
Nursing home	2.2	0.0	0.0
Totals	**40.3**	**35.3**	**24.8**
Phone calls (to/from)			
Patient/relative	4.4	4.0	9.6
Team/staff/providers	7.1	6.4	18.3
Totals	**11.5**	**10.4**	**27.9**
Administration			
Record writing	9.1	11.3	14.9
Clinical conference	4.1	7.3	7.3
Other *	14.6	13.2	11.4
Totals	**27.8**	**31.8**	**33.6**
Travel	20.7	31.2	20.1

* Nontelephone interactions with providers, administrators, relatives, etc.

outside home care. I am led to believe the Rochester data, shown in Table 2.3, is based on 10 years' experience with a similar team.

Patient contact time per visit was 39 minutes for physicians, 49 minutes for nurse practitioners, and 70 minutes for social workers. The authors felt that 1 physician, working with 1.5 nurse practitioners and 1 social worker, could meet the medical home care needs of 100 such patients. This intensive staffing ratio implies either very difficult cases or inefficient providers. Consider, however, NH, a 79-year-old woman who has lived for years with severe, steroid-dependent asthma, widespread osteoarthritis, venous thromboembolic disease on chronic warfarin, osteoporosis, spinal stenosis, heart disease, and anxiety. Though sedentary, she lived alone, worried about her health, and periodically visited the emergency room for asthma or chest pain.

Then she noticed a little blood coming from either her rectum or vagina. On examination there was a trace of blood in her rectum, and her uterus was enlarged. She wanted to be sure she did not have cancer. To proceed meant sigmoidoscopy and possibly pelvic ultrasound or uterine biopsy. Two specialists would be consulted, tests would be scheduled, and several ambulance rides would be arranged. The specialists would need to understand NH's frail medical condition to guide their evaluation and recommendations. Care coordination involves a lot of time.

Before applying care management time to my Richmond practice, consider that our patients average 10 house calls per year, each house call averaging 1 hour, including travel. Some patients are seen twice yearly for maintenance care; others are seen 30 times for both acute and chronic problems. This average visit frequency approximates that for nursing home patients and ambulatory frail elders (see chapter 9), which seem reasonable benchmarks. Adding 40% for care management brings us from 10 to 14 hours per patient each year. Given 21 such patients in a practice, they would consume 294 hours annually, or 6 hours in a 60-hour week. A few patients can command 10% of one's time.

Compare this with weekly home care management time reported in the 1990 physician survey.[48] As shown in Table 2.4, the analysis separated physicians into three groups by frequency of their referrals to home health agencies. Questions were phrased as follows: "During a typical week, how many hours do you spend managing home care by phone?" and "During a typical week, how many hours do you spend completing forms related to home care?" The data were grouped by 1-hour intervals, most responses falling in the 0–1-hour, 1–2-hour, or 2–3-hour categories. Combining all respondents, the average weekly home care efforts were 2.1 hours on the phone and 1.5 hours on paperwork.

The survey is admittedly imprecise. For example, the increase in care management time for physicians in the high-referral group is not proportionate to the increase in homebound patients and referrals. The discrepancy is too great to represent learning curve effects. Yet the averages for the intermediate group and for the total sample are generally consistent with my earlier care management work estimates. Respondents with 19 homebound patients reported 3 to 4 hours of care management. The main difference between their practices and mine or the Rochester team's appears to be the low house call frequency. And the 1990 national survey's imprecision, compared with the more precise time-motion study, is balanced by a far broader representation of physician practices.

TABLE 2.4 Annual Home Care Referral Frequency

General characteristic	Low (0–11 referrals) (N=429)	Intermediate (12–47 referrals) (N=417)	High (>47 referrals) (N=315)
Total work hr/wk	60	62	65
Patient care hr/wk	52	55	57
Number of homebound	12	19	36
Number of referrals/yr	3	24	95
Number of house calls/yr	7	8	12
Home care management			
Phone work hrs/wk	1.4	2.1	2.6
Paperwork hrs/wk	1.2	1.3	2.1

From "A National Survey of the Home Visiting Practice & Attitudes of Family Physicians & Internists," by Keenan et al., 1992, *Archives of Internal Medicine, 40*, 1241–1249. Copyright © 1994, by Williams & Wilkins. Reprinted with permission.

The low house call frequency is also understandable. Time, money, schedules, and efficiency are critical for practicing physicians. The Rochester and MCV Home Care teams are partially sheltered by external financial support. Like community physicians, my medical center colleagues find house calls difficult to schedule, too costly of time, and too poorly reimbursed. I suspect that the amount of time practicing physicians commit to care of the homebound is less than many would recommend when designing an ideal care delivery system, but busy physicians balancing priorities must find themselves postponing something. Urgent clinical problems and patient requests, most originating in offices and hospitals, have pressing immediacy. It is conceivable that lower priority might be accorded to completing insurance forms, making nursing home rounds or house calls, or doing home care paperwork. As care delivery systems evolve and coalesce around community needs, we should see better approaches to delivery and coordination of home care (see chapter 8).

PREPARING FOR MEDICAL CARE
IN A HOME SETTING

One reason given for not making house calls is the belief that physicians cannot give adequate care at home. The 1990 national survey[1] showed that 61% of physicians who make house calls and 42% of those who do not make house calls agreed with the statement: "I can provide adequate medical care in the home." Adelman reported similar data from a large national mail survey of primary care physicians.[49] Among physicians who did not make house calls or who had stopped making house calls, concern about inability to provide the "usual quality of care" was endorsed by 76% of family physicians, 81% of internists, and 89% of pediatricians.

From my experience, this perception is usually inaccurate. Almost any service provided in a physician's office can be provided at home by experienced and properly equipped home care physicians. Most services offered in emergency rooms can be delivered in most Richmond homes. Here's an example of what we routinely do.

I saw WW as a new patient one day at 4 P.M. He was a large man, totally paralyzed on the right side and unable to speak after a stroke, who lived on the second floor of his own house with his wife. He could travel only by ambulance, so his wife was very grateful for the house call. Coincidentally, WW was sick that afternoon, having suffered diarrhea and abdominal pain for 2 days. In the past this had caused an ileus, a partial paralysis of bowel function due to low blood potassium levels, and he was then hospitalized for 2 weeks.

I examined WW under the bright sunlight from his bedroom window. He appeared uncomfortable but not acutely ill, yet his abdomen was swollen tight as a drum. Based on the high-pitched tinkles, gurgles, and rushes coming through my stethoscope, another ileus appeared imminent. My office-based home care coordinator arranged an abdominal X-ray while I drew some blood. The X-ray crew arrived with their portable equipment before I left. They were sweating after carrying this load up the stairs, but it was far easier than carrying WW down!

Within 2 hours I was paged and given the test results. The X ray showed colonic pseudo-obstruction, and the labs revealed a very low potassium level, but no other serious problems. I had WW's phone number. A local pharmacy, a few blocks from WW's home, was closing as I called. This pharmacist is a compassionate man with whom we work closely. He waited a few minutes so that WW's wife could pick up the potassium her husband needed. Two days later he was fine.

In Richmond, I am fortunate to have portable X-ray and ECG services that are not available in rural areas. Still, we need such services for only a fraction of our housecalls. More frequently needed is laboratory support: some diagnostic test follows one-third of our visits. We obtain specimens and transport them to the hospital for processing. If urgent, we have lab results in a few hours. X-ray and ECG reports are equally rapid. A complete evaluation can easily be done within half a workday and we are often as fast as our understaffed and overloaded emergency room.

Even more rapid urgent care can be obtained by consolidating the clinical team, lab, and radiology services in a mobile unit. Although ideally suited to urgent care, and more efficient in such cases, such mobile units carry more equipment and more overhead than is needed for most house calls. However, future widespread use of the compact portable lab devices now available is inevitable once a few technical issues are resolved and the Clinical Laboratories Improvement Amendment of 1988 (CLIA) bureaucracy is addressed.

Other lab work is obtained for us by visiting nurses. They use private laboratories whose runners pick up specimens from several "drops." Same-day service is available, often for an extra fee, but most results return the following day. This system is slower and more cumbersome than using our hospital laboratory, and it is far slower than the on-site portable lab. Private lab technicians will also visit patients to draw blood, also involving a fee and slow turn-around. Nationwide, most home care lab work is currently handled by nursing agencies and commercial or hospital-based labs. The use of new portable technologies will greatly enhance the efficiency of lab support for home care.

Soon I may carry a miniature lab on my house calls, yet even now I carry a more modern equivalent of the old-time doctor's black bag. Mine is a green medium-sized overnight bag with a shoulder strap, and it contains these items:

- Sphygmomanometer (blood pressure measurement device with hand-held gauge) and several cuffs, including a thigh cuff.
- Battery-powered kit for ear, eye, nose, and throat exams.
- Thermometers with disposable covers (electronic thermometers; mercury boils if left too long in the car under the hot summer sun, ruining a glass thermometer).

- Basic wound dressings: (4 x 4 gauze, tape, gloves, iodine, 3-inch Kling gauze).
- Wound debridement supplies (gloves, scalpel, disposable debridement sets, sutures, a new bottle of local anesthetic).
- Rectal exam/disimpaction supplies (gloves, stool guaiac cards, lubricant).
- Urinary catheter supplies (disposable catheterization kit, catheters, specimen bottles).
- Fishing tackle box with venipuncture supplies (tourniquets, needles, syringes, alcohol pads, specimen tubes, gauze), injectable furosemide, and steroids for joint injections.
- Approved "sharps" disposal container.
- Cooler for lab specimens (summertime item).
- Industrial strength toenail clippers and safety goggles (acquired after a nurse practitioner caught a toenail chip in the eye, which proved a fairly serious injury).
- Nasogastric tubes and one empty tube feeding bag.
- Glucometer (optional).

Planning ahead is important. It is frustrating and inefficient to find unexpected problems that require a second visit after fetching the needed tools. Our bags were stocked by trial and error and some items are carried only for specific cases. For example, skin biopsies are done rarely and are planned, so we carry the biopsy device and fixative for that visit only. We have portable scales. If patients can stand, have no scale, and are being monitored for conditions like heart failure where weight is often the best indicator of therapeutic effect, a scale joins the day's baggage.

Even with this basic equipment, advanced medical treatment can be delivered at home. One Thursday I went to drain OD's boil. She was usually seen by my partner, who spends Thursdays at the nursing home, and OD's nurse practitioner was out sick. OD's relative called that morning to report a boil developing under the arm for several days, now the size of a "fifty-cent piece." My late afternoon schedule was open for coverage. I made OD's house call my last professional task for the day.

OD became bedfast after a stroke paralyzed her left side and affected her judgment. Her right arm remained powerful and she could speak clearly. As I approached the bed, she made a fist and said, "Goddamit! Leave me alone. If you touch me, I'll hit you." I asked what was wrong. She said she had a boil. I looked at the angry, fluctuant boil, 2 inches across and nearly an inch deep, visible below her right armpit and told her it required drainage. She said she wanted a boil plaster. Two middle-aged ladies, her relatives and caregivers, told OD she would have no choice. The boil would be drained.

My bag was set on a nearby table, which became a procedure stand. With OD's right arm pinioned by a loving relative who sang to her, the abscess was prepped with iodine, anesthetized, incised, drained, probed, irrigated, packed, and dressed. Paper towels prevented staining the bedclothes and nightshirt. As I finished, I ran out of adhesive tape. One lady went across the street to her house and returned with some Band-aids. We made a satisfactory though unorthodox dressing from my gauze and her Band-aids. I ordered antibiotics by phone, which another relative was sent to buy. The whole process took less than an hour. Friday I would arrange home nursing for wound care.

Protesting the indignity of her position throughout the procedure, at one point OD said, "I want to go to the hospital!" Her cousin responded, "Why do you want to go to the hospital? Everything they have there we have right here." I endorse that opinion and add that we gained additional benefits by performing the surgery at home, not the least of which was a team of friendly helpers with familiar faces to restrain OD's powerful right arm. A group of young children watching also began the cultural transformation required to bring physicians back to the home. Later, OD thanked me for helping her. She capped the visit by telling me to send a big nurse. Asked why, she made a fist and answered, "Otherwise, I'll knock her down," continuing to assert her fierce desire for control over her life.

Based on my experience and assuming the proper preparation and support, I join the 61% of house call physicians in our national telephone survey who felt that high-quality medical care can be delivered at home. With this, I turn in chapter 3 to relationships between physicians and other home care professionals.

REFERENCES

1. Keenan JM, Boling PA, Schwartzberg JG, Olson L, Schneidermann M, McCaffrey DJ, Ripsin CM. A national survey of the home visiting practice and attitudes of family physicians and internists. *Arch Intern Med.* 1992; 152:2025–2032.
2. Col N, Fanale JE, Kronholm P. The role of medication noncompliance and adverse drug reactions in the elderly. *Arch Intern Med.* 1990; 150:841–845.

3. Hanlon J, Weinberger M, Samsa G, Schmader K, Uttech K, Lewis I, Cowper P, Landsman P, Feussner J, Cohen HJ. A randomized controlled trial of a clinical pharmacist intervention for elderly outpatients with polypharmacy. *J Am Geriatr Soc.* 1994; 42 (11): Abstract A24.

4. Sullivan DH, Walls RC. Impact of nutritional status on morbidity in a population of geriatric rehabilitation patients. *J Am Geriatr Soc.* 1994; 42:471–477.

5. Drickamer MA, Cooney LM. A geriatrician's guide to enteral feeding. *J Am Geriatr Soc.* 1993; 41:672–679.

6. Strauss MJ, Gong J, Gary BD, Kalsbeek WD, Spear S. The cost of home air-fluidized therapy for pressure sores: A randomized controlled trial. *J Fam Pract.* 1991; 33(1):52–59.

7. Ferrell BA, Keeler E, Siu AL, Ahn SH, Osterweil D. Cost-effectiveness of low-air-loss beds in nursing homes. *J Am Geriatr Soc.* 1994; 42: 41.

8. Simon A. Some observations of a geropsychiatrist on the value of housecalls. *Gerontologist.* 1984; 24(5):458–464.

9. Muijen M, Marks I, Connolly J, Audini B. Home based care and standard care for patients with severe mental illness: A randomized controlled trial. *Br Med J.* 1992; 304:749–754.

10. Dean C, Phillips J, Gadd EM, Joseph M, England S. Comparison of community based service with hospital based service for people with acute, severe psychiatric illness. *Br Med J.* 1993; 307:473–464.

11. Spiro AH. Psychiatric home care: A new tool for crisis intervention. *Newsletter of the American Academy of Home Care Physicians.* 1993; 5(3):10.

12. Bruce ML, McNamara R. Psychiatric status among the homebound elderly: An epidemiologic perspective. *J Am Geriatr Soc.* 1992; 40:561–566.

13. Series F, Marc I, Cormier Y, La Forge J. Utility of nocturnal home oximetry for case finding in patients with suspected sleep apnea syndrome. *Ann Intern Med.* 1993; 119(6):449–453.

14. Moss AH, Casey P, Stocking CB, Roos RP, Brooks BR, Siegler M. Home ventilation for amyotrophic lateral sclerosis patients: Outcomes, costs, and patient, family, and physician attitudes. *Neurology.* 1993; 43(2):438–443; 1993.

15. Senders CW, Muntz HR, Schweiss D. Physician survey of the care of children with tracheostomy. *Am J Otolaryngology.* 1991; 12(1):48–50.

16. Ford C, Iliffe S, Franklin O. Outcome of planned home births in an inner city practice. *Br Med J.* 1991; 303:1517–1519.

17. US Preventive Services Task Force releases policy statement on home uterine activity monitoring. *Am Fam Physician.* 1993; 48(5):932–935.

18. Gordon M, Cheung M. Poor outcome of on-site CPR in a multi-level geriatric facility: Three and a half years' experience at the Baycrest Center for Geriatric Care. *J Am Geriatr Soc.* 1993; 41:163–166.

19. Rhiner M, Ferrell BR, Ferrell BA, Grant MM. A structured nondrug inter-

vention program for cancer pain. *Cancer Practice.* 1993; 1(2):137–143.

20. Thorpe G. Enabling more dying people to remain at home. *Br Med J.* 1993; 307:915–918.

21. Rosenbaum EH, Rosenbaum IR. Principles of home care for the patient with advanced cancer. *JAMA.* 1980; 244(13):1484–1487.

22. Rosenblatt DE, Campion EW, Mason M. Rehabilitation home visits. *J Am Geriatr Soc.* 1986; 34:441–447.

23. Portnow J. ed., Home health care and rehabilitation. *Physical Medicine and Rehabilitation.* 1988; 2(3):279–465.

24. Parver C. Certificates of medical necessity for home medical equipment: What physicians need to know. *American Academy of Home Care Physicians Newsletter.* 1994; 6(2):5–6.

25. Reuben DB, Zwanziger J, Bradley TB, Beck JC. Is geriatrics a primary care or subspecialty discipline? *J Am Geriatr Soc.* 1994; 42(4):363–367.

26. Mahmud K, Keenan JM, Bennett MB. Home heparin infusion in the management of deep vein thrombophlebitis. *Minnesota Medicine.* 1990; 73:31–33.

27. Sternberg S. *Medical Economics.* June 13, 1994; 16–127.

28. Outpatient use of intravenous antibiotics. Poretz DM, guest editor. *Am J Med.* 1994; 97(2A):1–55.

29. Tice AD. Outpatient parenteral antibiotic therapy: Part 2. *Hosp Pract.* 1993; 28(suppl 2):5–64.

30. Detsky AS, McLaughlin JR, Abrams HB, L'Abbe KA, Whitwell J, Bombardier C, Jeejeebhoy KN. Quality of life of patients on long-term total parenteral nutrition at home. *J Gen Intern Med.* 1986; 1:26–33.

31. Power EJ. Home drug infusion therapy under Medicare. *JAMA.* 1993; 270(4):427.

32. New PB, Swanson GF, Bulich RG, Taplin GC. Ambulatory antibiotic infusion devices: Extending the spectrum of outpatient therapies. *Am J Med.* 1991; 91:455–461.

33. Koopman MMW, Prandoni P, Piovella F, et al. Treatment of venous thrombosis with intravenous unfractionated heparin administered in the hospital as compared with subcutaneous low-molecular-weight heparin administered at home. *N Engl J Med.* 1996; 334(11):682–687.

34. Levine M, Gent M, Hirsh J, et al. A comparison of low-molecular-weight heparin administered primarily at home with unfractionated heparin administered in the hospital for proximal deep-vein thrombosis. *N Engl J Med.* 1996; 334(11):677–681.

35. Lawson M, Bottino JC, et al. The use of urokinase to restore the patency of occluded central venous catheters. *American Journal of Intravenous Therapy and Clinical Nutrition.* 1982; 29–32.

36. Rawles J. Halving of mortality at 1 year by domiciliary thrombolysis in the Grampian Region Early Antistreplase Trial (GREAT). *J Am Coll Cardiol.* 1994; 23:1–5.

37. Goldberg AI, Monahan CA. Home health care for children assisted by mechanical ventilation: The physician's perspective. *J Pediatr.* 1989; 114:378–383.

38. Schreiner MS, Downes JJ, Kettrick RG, Ise C, Voit R. Chronic respiratory failure in infants with prolonged ventilator dependency. *JAMA.* 1987; 258:3398–3404.

39. Frates RC, Splaingard ML, Smith EO, Harrison GM. Outcome of home mechanical ventilation in children. *J Pediatr.* 1985; 106:850–856.

40. Fischer JR, Kaatz BL. Continuous subcutaneous infusion of terbutaline for suppression of preterm labor. Clin Pharm. 1991; 10:292–296.

41. Meropol SB, Luberti AA, De Jong AR, Weiss JC. Home phototherapy: Use and attitudes among community pediatricians. *Pediatrics.* 1993; 91:97–100.

42. Cauthen DB. The house call in current medical practice. *J Fam Pract.* 1981; 13(2):209–213.

43. Burton JR. The house call: An important service for the frail elderly. *J Am Geriatr Soc.* 1985; 33:291–293.

44. Siwek J. House calls: Current status and rationale. *Am Fam Physician.* 1985; 31(4):169–174.

45. Knight AL, Adelman AM. The family physician and home care. *Am Fam Phys.* 1991; 44:1733–1737.

46. Gonzalez ML, ed. *Socioeconomic Characteristics of Medical Practice 1990/ 1991.* Chicago, IL: Center for Health Policy Research, American Medical Association; 1991.

47. Zimmer JG, Groth-Juncker A. A time-motion study of patient care activities of a geriatric home care team. *Home Health Care Services Quarterly.* 1983; 4(1):67–78.

48. Boling PA, Keenan JM, Schwartzberg JS, Retchin SM, Olson L, Schneiderman M. Reported home health agency referrals by internists and family physicians. *J Am Geriatr Soc.* 1992; 40:1241–1249.

49. Adelman AM, Fredman L, Knight AL. House call practices: A comparison by specialty. *J Fam Pract.* 1994; 39(1):39–44.

CHAPTER 3

Home Care Physicians and the Interdisciplinary Team

I n the last chapter, I described the type of work done by the physician as a home care provider. In this chapter, I will discuss working relationships between physicians and the core members of an interdisciplinary home care team that delivers most of the professional home care. This area of home care urgently needs focused attention and energy in the next few years,

HOME CARE PHYSICIANS WORKING IN A TEAM ENVIRONMENT

Whether they work in busy office practices or mobile home care units, physicians whose signatures authorize home health services are members of a team. A 1990 national survey[1] showed that physicians spend substantial time on home care management. Yet other data show the need for more active physician participation,[2] and conversations with thousands of home health agency workers tell of great variation in physician commitment. In fact, many physicians are seen by home health agencies and home equipment vendors as inaccessible, ill-informed about home care, and slow to comply with regulatory requirements such as completing and signing forms. It is felt that some physicians avoid using home care for fear that this will reduce visits to their offices. Some agency staff also feel that physicians are too reluctant to relinquish control over patients' care.

On the other side, physicians report that home health personnel do not understand physicians' needs, needlessly interrupt them with nonurgent phone calls, and deluge them with paperwork that is bureaucratic and nonclinical. Inconsistent quality of home health agency services is another issue. Finally, physicians have felt they are not compensated for their work supporting home care, whereas agencies are paid well for providing services.

Obviously, this picture of physicians and home health care workers doesn't describe a match made in heaven. Yet many physicians who are community-oriented and experienced in home care have excellent relationships with home health agencies and equipment companies. What makes the relationship work?

First is commonality of purpose. The common goal must be to optimize outcomes for patient and caregivers. This automatically puts both parties on the same team. Second is mutual understanding and respect. Both parties must understand each other's realities, competencies, and limitations. Each must respect the other's ability to contribute in caring for the patient. I find that understanding and respect come from seeing the world where the other person lives and works and from seeing what the other person can accomplish. Third, and perhaps most important, is communication. This cannot be emphasized enough, and several strategies discussed below have proved useful in fostering good communication.

Team relationships are common in many medical settings. The smallest office practice usually includes a physician, nurse, and receptionist, who work side by side every day. If they do not communicate well and work together, the practice fails. Team connections are less tight on inpatient wards, where rotating shifts of nurses and other staff collaborate with attending physicians who visit the ward and direct care. Physicians count on staff to conduct most of the care, enact their orders, make independent assessments and judgments, and communicate effectively. Physicians often know the strengths, weaknesses, and styles of staff on the wards they frequent, and the staff learn the physicians' idiosyncrasies and capabilities. Like home care, much of inpatient care is ordered by telephone or computer. Similar team situations are found in intensive care units, emergency rooms, operating rooms, recovery rooms, and delivery rooms. All of these teams tend to have far stronger linkages than home care teams. Home care team linkages must improve.

MAKING THE TEAM WORK BETTER

An event common to these other settings and rare in home care is the team visit. By this I mean a visit involving multiple disciplines. Beside the camaraderie that this usually creates, I know several justifications for occasionally incurring the operational expense of a home care team visit. Because of the cost and logistic complexity of coordinating efforts, however, we carefully select the circumstances for all such team visits.

For instance, one circumstance indicating that a team visit may be needed is a difficult, unresolved social situation. Gathering the family, physician, social worker, and nurse or nurse practitioner in one room ensures that all parties hear the same dialogue, that professionals with diverse skills are present to address the various aspects of the problem, and that, if necessary, the professional team presents a strong and unified front to induce changes in caregiver or patient behavior. Medical information gathering and decision making are additional indications for a team visit. I periodically make joint visits with nurses, nurse practitioners, or physical therapists to confirm physical findings, give advice about managing a specific problem, or learn from them about my patient's condition and needs.

Two other considerations are safety and efficiency. So far, Richmond has not proved dangerous for daytime house calls. However, there are localities, usually in the poverty zones of large cities or in some isolated rural areas, where there is greater safety in numbers. And efficiency can actually be enhanced by team visits. For example, the nurse can start the wound care while I interview the family or examine the patient's heart. When the wounds are exposed, the nurse and I can confer about wound care options and medical management. I can leave while the nurse dresses the wound. If I were alone, I would have to undo and later restore the nurse's dressing to assess the wound, thus inefficiently performing redundant work.

Besides team visits there are many other strategies that may improve home care team functioning. One is to limit the size of the team. Generally, the more often team members interact, the more familiar they become with each other's needs and habits and the more efficient the team becomes. Thus, it may be helpful to limit the number of home care agencies and the number of individual agency personnel with whom a given physician interacts. Using preferred providers can facilitate team building and communication.

Another good strategy is the team meeting. Some physicians with large home care practices have regularly scheduled care management conferences with home health agency staff. Many home-based health care (HBHC) programs at Veterans Affairs hospitals use this model. The core staff of Medical College of Virginia (MCV) Home Care (physicians, nurse practitioners, social worker, and patient advocate) meet weekly. For years we have also met monthly with staff from the Instructive Visiting Nurse Association (IVNA), which handles the home health agency care for most of our patients.

Despite the linkage with the IVNA, the number of nurses with whom we worked was initially too great. Continuity of nursing care, familiarity of the nurses with MCV Home Care operations, comfort of MCV Home Care staff with the nurses' skills, and communication were all suboptimal. Imagine a physician's office having different nurses every few days! We now work with a subunit of the IVNA, and the teamwork is smoother. During monthly meetings, we discuss clinical problems, keep notes that document care management, sign forms, and resolve process problems that hinder the interface between MCV Home Care and the IVNA.

Though MCV Home Care staff don't meet regularly with other home health allies, like medical equipment providers or pharmacists, such meetings are an option. Still, we have working relationships with selected equipment providers, one of two local mobile X-ray services, pharmacies that deliver, and other community resources. Again, these relationships are not exclusive, but when we have a difficult case or a situation needing a reliable, friendly response, there is a short list of people we usually call, and they handle most of our business. In general, as these relationships become tighter, the process of care becomes more efficient.

For most physicians, particularly those with small home care practices, scheduled meetings or preferred provider relationships may be impractical. Yet specific strategies to improve team function are still vital. One common problem is "telephone tag," which causes enormous waste and inefficiency in home care. Here is the too familiar scenario. A nurse sees a patient at home and calls the doctor's office for new orders. The doctor is with a patient. When the doctor is free and calls the agency, the nurse is at another home and the agency's office staff doesn't know exactly what the nurse needed. All parties are frustrated, care is delayed, and time is wasted.

COMMUNICATING EFFECTIVELY
WITH OTHER TEAM MEMBERS

One solution to phone tag is for physicians and home health providers to designate specific times and methods for nonurgent consultation and to define in advance a plan for urgent contact (e.g., pager, fax, or a specific contact person). At the agency, nurses must develop some type of message drop, normally involving an office-based nurse. This person must know what the field nurse wishes to communicate to the physician. Further enhancing the interaction, nurses may be assisted by standardized tools so that messages to physicians are complete, reducing the need for additional calls. Consider a patient taking warfarin, an anticoagulant that interacts with numerous other medicines plus some foods and physiological processes and thus necessitating close monitoring of a blood test (INR) and frequent dose adjustments. Possible consequences of inattention can include fatal hemorrhage or thromboembolism, so the stakes are high. In addition to the INR value, the physician deciding about medication changes needs to know about the patient's current medication dose, compliance, diet, status of heart and liver functions, signs of excessive bleeding, and any recent addition or deletion of other medicines. If this standardized dataset came with a flow sheet of recent INR values and dose changes, telephone management of warfarin at home would be simplified and improved.

Unfortunately, this vital interface issue has not been resolved in most home care practices, and it must become a top priority for all home care providers. Ultimately, communication will further improve with new information technology such as voice mail, electronic mail, or electronic medical records. (See section in chapter 8).

OTHER PROBLEMS TEAMS FACE

Fostering Dependency

Patients who come to the office assume some responsibility for their care by so doing. In chronic home care, patients and caregivers can become too dependent on professionals. One manifestation is the tendency to call about minor problems, without trying to assess the situation. Dependency is not unique to home care, as any primary care physician knows, but perhaps dependency is found more often in home care because so much care is given by informal caregivers, who are caring for vulnerable relatives and are uncertain about the meaning of changes in clinical status. Fortunately, pathological dependency is relatively rare.

Occasionally, home care also can foster immobility by removing one more reason for frail patients to mobilize and leave home. This is concern is often overemphasized. Truly homebound patients visit physician offices infrequently, and sorties from the home don't provide much physical activity. A few patients gain psychological benefit from going to see their physicians. Making it to the office may be a matter of pride and proof of functional capability. This opportunity should not be denied when patients want it.

Waiting Too Long

This is a slight variation on the theme discussed above. The danger can be manifested in two ways. One is when caregivers count on professionals to detect all new problems that may develop. This is a particular concern for patients who are seen at home frequently and whose caregivers lack medical sophistication. The second arises when home care is used to manage serious, acute problems like pneumonia, complicated urinary tract infections, dehydration, electrolyte abnormalities, deep vein thrombosis, stroke, or myocardial infarction. Acute home care can be highly appropriate and effective. However, some patients require hospitalization for optimal outcomes. Even though goals may shift from cure to comfort when the overall prognosis is poor and hospitalization increases the risk of iatrogenic illness,[3] it is possible to wait too long, with undesirable consequences. Experience greatly improves the chances of making wise choices in these cases, as there are no formal guidelines or empiric studies on which to lean.

INSUFFICIENT PHYSICIAN HOUSE CALLS

It is also obvious that physicians on home care teams need to make some house calls to be effective team members. In other clinical settings, physicians don't order or direct medical care from a distance, even on the recommendation of other skilled professionals, unless they know the staff and the patient very well. Why should home care be different? What happens when physicians are not actively involved? In the end some patients with reversible problems unnecessarily enter nursing homes, emergency room and hospital costs increase, medical decisions suffer, and quality of care diminishes.

THE HOME CARE PHYSICIAN AS CONSULTANT
OR ADMINISTRATOR

There is a growing trend to recruit physicians as medical directors of home health agencies or as consultants. In 1990, 13% of internists and family physicians had served as home health agency medical directors, on the boards of home health agencies, or as home care consultants.[4] This is an important development. A physician who is knowledgeable about home care and dedicated to the process can enhance an agency's service delivery and form an important bridge to other physicians. The full potential of this physician home care role has not yet been realized, even though the value of medical direction was recognized early in the home care renaissance of the 1970s. However, unlike nursing homes, home health agencies are not required to have medical directors, and only a fraction of agencies have them. Smaller agencies often find the cost insupportable. Others note that the role has been fulfilled inconsistently; many medical directors perform brief infrequent, perfunctory administrative services. Finally, there is a shortage of physicians qualified for this role.

The shortage is now being addressed by a 20-hour workshop created by the American Academy of Home Care Physicians. Taking cues from the nursing home medical director experience, we borrowed from a well-developed literature[5] and curricula offered by the American Medical Directors Association. After surveying a group of home care agency medical directors, we held a focus group at the academy's 1995 annual meeting, later followed by two intensive workshop planning sessions. The result was an interactive workshop in which communication and teamwork skills were emphasized while covering the key subject matter, as shown in Table 3.1. Feedback from both physicians and agencies has been very positive.

There are three final considerations about the medical advisor role. One is that fully developing the home care agency medical director work force

TABLE 3.1 AAHCP Home Health Agency Medical Director Workshop Content

Utilization review and quality improvement	Developing new services and strategic planning
Educational programs and in-services for staff development	Occupational medicine and employee health
Community liaison, particularly with other physicians	Medical and professional ethical issues
Compliance with regulatory standards	Health services research applications

will take time. Recall that despite great strides and years of work, performance by nursing home medical directors still varies widely.[6,7] Second, in addition to traditional agency medical direction, large national home care companies and managed care delivery systems are employing physicians as consultants, to guide performance improvement, integration of physician and agency services, and other activities that enhance home care teamwork. Finally, there is the 1993 Stark legislation (Medicare Conditions of Payment. 42 U.S.C. & 1395f(a); 42 U.S.C. & 424.24(d)(2) & 424.24(d)(3) that limits the compensation, not just salary, a physician may receive from an agency serving that physician's patients to 5% of the agency's operating expenses, or $25,000, whichever is less. Thus, a physician who spends a substantial amount of time as a paid medical director often cannot refer patients to that agency.

THE PROFESSIONAL CARE
PROVIDER WORK FORCE

A valuable resource that has been underutilized in home care is the professional care provider. Generally speaking, I refer here to nurse practitioners and physician assistants, though clinical nurse specialists and nurse midwifes also have a role. The remainder of this chapter will explore the potential of these providers to enhance home care teams.

Several new professional provider disciplines, with diagnostic and therapeutic capabilities intermediate between registered nurses and physicians, originated in the 1970s. These providers are recognized as a valuable resource,[8] even though full recognition of their value is still lacking.[9] I will review some of the data supporting the role of care providers, much of it now decades old. The evidence is strong, yet the slow evolution of our practices speaks to the influence of tradition. Despite these slow beginnings the practicing cohort and the number of new graduates in the professional care provider disciplines is now sizable and growing. Precise work force estimates are hindered by lack of uniform standards and central registries. For example, new nurse practitioners now receive master's degrees, but many of those currently licensed graduated from certificate programs. Some of these were retraining programs that offered less intensive curricula than those of current programs. Still there are now at least 35,000 active nurse practitioners and 32,000 physician assistants.

The distribution of this work force is also important because these professionals have been seen as one answer to provider shortages in underserved areas and primary care fields. This vision has not been entirely fulfilled. Yankauer and Sullivan[10] noted that 75% of nurse practitioners and physician assistants entered primary care practice by 1980, but relatively few were located in underserved areas, which today still remain underserved. In 1993 the American Academy of Physician Assistants reported that 17% of physician assistants practiced in towns of under 10,000, and 45% worked with primary care physicians. Demand for professional care providers remains high, but there are marked state-to-state variations in the numbers of active professional care providers, suggesting regional differences in training or acceptance of the role. And regarding gerontologic nurse practitioners (GNPs), Ebersole[11] noted that 23,600 nursing homes housed 1.5 million residents, yet approximately 250 nursing homes had a GNP on staff, while 350 GNPs were doing teaching and research work.

EFFECT OF PROFESSIONAL CARE PROVIDERS ON PHYSICIAN PRACTICES

In settings shared with physicians, care providers substitute for physicians to varying degrees, depending on how the practice is organized, the capabilities and preferences of providers and patients, and the nature of patients' problems. The numbers of patients seen by professional care providers each day and the proportionate practice expansion thus generated depend on the practice's organization. If they provide telephone support rather than seeing patients, care providers' visit volumes may be lower. However, in a managed care situation, increasing office visits does not always bring success. Efficiency of care measured by cost per episode of illness rather than by number of visits was shown to be greater when nurse practitioners were included.[12] Similarly, analyzing efficiency by aggregate value of services produced (26% increase) rather than by visits (6% increase) casts a more favorable light on the impact of professional care providers.[13]

These providers have a variety of roles. The 1980 Graduate Medical Education National Advisory Committee (GMENAC) report on professional care providers noted typical rates, when substituting care providers for physicians, that ranged between 8% and 48% of visits, depending on the complaint. And a 1985 study of three practice models found actual substitution rates varying from 1% to 70%.[14]

Several studies have examined the effect of professional care providers on ambulatory practices. One early study of MEDEX providers (military medics retrained to be physician assistants) showed a 37% increase in office visits.[15] In the well-designed Burlington randomized trial, physician practices utilizing nurse practitioners were compared to practices without nurse practitioners. Clinical quality ratings, patient outcomes, and patient satisfaction were similar. Once roles and relationships were established, nurse practitioners were able to manage two-thirds of office visits without consultation.[16,17] This was based on encounters rather than patients. I remind readers that although a given patient may have numerous encounters that do not require the physician, when the patient does need the physician, it is best that the physician and the patient know one another.

FINANCIAL IMPACTS OF PROFESSIONAL CARE PROVIDERS ON PHYSICIAN PRACTICES

The financial effect of professional care providers on physician practices was deemed complex by the Office of Technology Assessment.[8] Expert opinions range from highly favorable to pessimistic. One advocate used mathematical models to estimate that in 1991 failure to use nurse practitioners in primary care would cause approximately $6 billion to $9 billion of excess expenses.[18] Others have thought the gain in productivity might be as small as 20%, with only minimal gains in net income. Most recently, the marketplace has spoken. Managed care systems have advanced the role of professional care providers in ambulatory care, based in part on analyses like that of Record et al.[19]

The basic idea is that the salaries and training costs of these professionals are lower than those of physicians. With a shorter training period, the care providers can handle two-thirds of the typical problems of physician offices. Additionally, professionals may be more skilled than physicians in some functions, thus increasing the practice's service capability.

The Geisinger Clinic administration estimated that a physician assistant employed in a family practice would generate $72,077 in new revenues and overhead reduction.[20] In 1991 the breakdown for the new monies came from office services and lab tests ($51,707), nursing home practice ($14,400), and improved physician office productivity brought about by reducing physician nursing home work ($3,750). Overhead reduction was modest ($2,220). Nursing home visits numbered 400, and office visits numbered 1,675. The benefits to cardiovascular surgeons ($332,000, mostly from freedom to perform more surgery) and to urologists ($156,350, divided between overhead reduction and the opportunity to perform more surgery) were considerably larger.

Data have suggested differences in productivity between nurse practitioners and physician assistants. In one example, physicians had 19 to 21 visits per day, physician assistants saw 14 patients, and nurse practitioners saw 8. All of the professional care providers spent comparably little time on the phone, and the physician assistants spent 30 minutes longer engaged in direct patient care each day. Income per encounter was 12% higher for physician assistants. In part, this difference may have been due to the fact that nurse practitioners were providing more counseling services.[21] I believe that these professional care provider disciplines do not inherently differ in efficiency but that the training, expectations and practice roles vary.

There is good evidence that most, though not all, patients are well satisfied by care received from professional care providers. For example, independent interviews of 214 patients were conducted in a randomly selected sample of 400 families from a private practice that had added nurse practitioners, finding that over 85% would recommend the practice to friends, and only three people were specifically opposed to the nurse practitioners.[22] In an Iowa community of 25,000, a practice used by blue-collar workers studied its patients and found some uncertainty over the physician assistant role, but 78% of respondents were usually or always satisfied by the team approach, and only eight percent exclusively wanted to see the physician.[23] Finally, rural patients were nearly neutral regarding issues of differential competency between physicians and nurse practitioners when treating serious problems, and they strongly endorsed availability, convenience, and ability to handle "minor" health problems.[24]

In my own experience, most patients are pleased with care they receive from our office nurse practitioners, though some express concern if the interval between physician visits grows too long. Some office patients and some home care patients *prefer* to see the nurse practitioners, which I consider a mark of success in attracting excellent co-workers. Still, there are some patients who feel strongly about seeing physicians on most or all occasions, and a few have left my practice, feeling that they could not reach me easily enough or see me often enough.

There is also solid evidence showing that nurse specialists give high-quality care, compared with that of physicians in outpatient, acute care, and nursing home settings.[25,26] Hypertensive control can be equivalent or better in the hands of nurse practitioners.[27] Nurse endoscopists can perform flexible sigmoidoscopy for screening as accurately and safely as gastroenterologists can.[28] Nurse midwives provide good care to women, including inpatient work.[29] Professional care providers are effective in public clinics[30,31] and subspecialty practices.[32] In addition to the excellent Burlington study, where quality of professional care providers' outpatient care was comparable to physician care, solid studies in the 1970s showed that MEDEX providers gave high-quality care, including in rural settings.[33]

PROFESSIONAL CARE PROVIDERS AND NURSING HOME CARE

Nurse practitioners have also been shown effective in geriatrics and long-term care, which is particularly relevant to the idea of nurse practitioner home care. One 1977 descriptive report favored a physician–nurse practitioner team model for geriatric ambulatory, home, and nursing home care. Since then, two prospective trials have shown that nurse practitioner involvement is associated with beneficial outcomes for nursing home patients.

One study, conducted in 1985, was based on the Mountain States Health Corporation program, which gave specialized training to experienced nurses, then placed these GNPs back in nursing homes, often their original institutions. The study compared care process and patient outcomes in 30 nursing homes employing nurse practitioners with control facilities. Significantly improved quality of care was noted for diabetes, heart failure, feeding problems, new urinary incontinence, and acute confusion.[34] Physician visits were reduced, while increased use of restorative nursing and gait training and less use of restraints indicated better care. Functional status improved only slightly. Emergency room use didn't change, but hospital admissions and hospital days were reduced.[35]

Implementing the new role of nurse practitioners in the nursing home proved sometimes difficult.[36] The largest hurdles included physician attitudes, other nurses' attitudes, role confusion with the nurse practitioner as administrator rather than clinician, and insufficient time to accomplish objectives. These difficulties may have vitiated the program's impact on costs. Other than slightly reduced emergency hospital days for patients newly admitted to the home, compared with those of established patients, which was unchanged, the nurse practitioner program had no effect on overall costs.[37] Also, when GNPs fully realized a clinical role, they were more satisfied and more likely to remain in the role.

The Massachusetts study had a different design.[38] There, 16 medical groups used a model developed by the Urban Medical Group,[39] in which clinic-based nurse practitioners and physician assistants provided nursing home care for patients from neighborhood health centers. The study had a Medicaid waiver, with professional care providers and physicians paid at identical rates for services, and no limit on the number of visits per patient. The nurses were attached to the physician groups rather than to the 186 nursing homes involved, and the unit of analysis was the patient rather than the facility. Control subjects were selected from nonstudy facilities to avoid study contamination. Matching of controls to intervention subjects was based on duration of institutional care, prior medical costs, age, and sex and on nursing home characteristics such as bed size, location, and type of ownership.

Patients receiving nurse-provided care received more on-site medical attention and had improved quality scores for several tracer conditions, including heart failure, hypertension, and new-onset urinary incontinence. At two per month, nursing home visits per patient nearly doubled, with extensive substitution of nurse visits for physician visits. This rate was considered appropriate. Emergency hospital use was significantly reduced, and total costs were reduced slightly; but confidence intervals were wide, and the difference was not significant. The authors noted that most patients were "roll-overs," previously in the nursing home and perhaps less likely to benefit because much of the high-intensity care for nursing home patients follows soon after admission.

The results of these two large studies were favorable enough to support Medicare and Medicaid payment for nurse practitioner nursing home work in the 1989 Omnibus Budget Reconciliation Act (OBRA). Continued failure of physicians to fulfill nursing home responsibilities, averaging only 1 hour per week in nursing homes,[40] was also a driving force behind the legislation.

REGULATORY AND LEGAL CHANGES RELATING TO PROFESSIONAL PROVIDERS

Controversy over "independent" practice by nurse care providers has been reflected in legal processes surrounding practice and payment. This comes into focus with prescriptive authority. Most states (46/50) and the District of Columbia allow nurse practitioners to prescribe medicines under guidelines defined in contracts with supervising physicians.

Laws specific to professional care providers caring for special populations are a critical issue for long-term care, including home care. The series of changes is nicely summarized by the Physician Payment Review Commission.[41] In 1989, Medicare started paying for nurse practitioner services in nursing homes without requiring the presence of a physician; physician assistants were accorded similar authority in 1986. The 1989 law was based in part on outcomes research and the serious shortage of qualified medical providers able or willing to work in nursing homes. William Kavesh played a role in promoting the 1989 OBRA law. He described to me a harrowing story of chance meetings and convergence of shifting political currents that allowed the law to pass, reminding us of the complex political process governing new policies.[42] Home care work was included in the original language of the bill but was removed during the legislative process.

Federal law was earlier modified in 1977 (P.L. 95-210), allowing Medicare payment for nurse practitioner house calls in areas without home health agencies, plus Medicaid payment for house calls by family and pediatric nurse practitioners, at the discretion of each state. The Medicare benefit was later extended to all rural settings (OBRA 1990, P.L. 101-508) but not to urban underserved areas. Under this law nurse practitioners and clinical nurse specialists were for the first time allowed to bill Medicare directly. Previously, all payments were delivered to their employers. The payment rate was required to be lower than the physician's rate.

State Medicaid programs differ from Medicare in covering professional care provider work in both rural and urban areas. Most states allow care by all nurse practitioners, not just the family and pediatric nurse practitioners specified by federal law, and such care providers are usually paid at the same low rate as physicians. For example, MCV Home Care nurse practitioners and I are paid the same $32.10 for a Medicaid house call.

NURSE CARE PROVIDERS IN HOME CARE: ROLES AND WORK LOAD

The experience with nursing home work is useful when considering home care for patients with severe functional impairment. The homebound need medical attention similar to that given in nursing homes, and the number of homebound patients is far greater than the number of physicians available, trained, willing, or funded to give them care. Nurse providers could address some of this unmet need.

Professional care providers may also be uniquely qualified for this work. I consider the different orientations of physicians and nurse practitioners to be beneficial. Several studies show that nurse practitioners are more likely to teach patients about exercise, diet, and other nonmedical aspects of health. And a recent prospective trial showed that home geriatric assessment by nurse practitioners can be clearly cost-effective.[43] In home care our nurse practitioners often have greater skill with nutrition, wound care, physical rehabilitation, and helping families to cope with chronic illness. I ask the nurse practitioners for advice as often as they seek my medical counsel.

Published models of long-term care teams in which physicians and nurses work together offer a framework for caseload and staffing parameters. For instance, in 1994 the San Diego Kaiser nursing home care system had 35,000 Medicare enrollees spread over 1,000 square miles, with

420 patients from 15 physician offices in 59 nursing homes.[44] Twenty percent of the patients needed skilled care. Resources for managing care of the 420 patients averaged 4.5 nurse practitioners, 4 geriatricians (who had additional duties), and 1.5 clerical personnel. Physicians' nursing home caseload was 52 to 130 patients, and nurse practitioners followed 60 to 102 patients. The geriatricians also supported geriatric clinics, home care, and hospices. Nurse practitioners saw nursing home patients monthly on average, with physician visits every 2 months.

In 1977 the previously mentionned East Boston Neighborhood Health Center system followed another urban population. Primary care physicians worked with professional care providers in four clinics, plus nursing home, hospital, and home settings. There were 3,000 clinic patients, 358 nursing home patients, and 280 home care patients. A quarter of the nursing home cases were in skilled care. The ambulatory practice ratio was 1.7 physicians to 0.5 professional care providers. Nursing home care involved three professional care providers, carrying 120 to 130 patients, making 30 to 35 visits per week, supported by 0.3 physician equivalents. Home care used one physician equivalent with five professional care providers, plus a full complement of traditional home health services, including two social workers. Professional care providers' home care caseload was 40 to 50 patients, with 20 to 22 visits per week. Telephone consultation was needed 10% of the time. Physicians handled all hospital care, which came to 7,882 inpatient days per 1,000 patients per year.

In chapter 2, I referred to Zimmer and the Rochester Home Health Care Team, which carried a small census of 54 seriously ill patients. Team members had responsibilities outside home care. Based on experience plus a time-and-motion study, the authors concluded that 1 physician, 1 social worker, and 1.5 nurse practitioners could manage 100 such patients. In Rochester nurse practitioners focused on home care, spending only 7% of their time in the hospital and none in nursing homes.

PERSONAL OBSERVATION ON NURSE PROVIDERS AND HOME CARE

I have worked closely with 20 nurse practitioners since 1984 in settings that include my private office, the hospital's outpatient clinic, the inpatient wards, the emergency department, and home care. The home care role differs from the others. I will write about nurse practitioners but consider them members of the larger category of professional care providers. Physician assistants, clinical nurse specialists, and nurse midwives all have potential importance for home care.

The MCV Home Care Program was established in 1986 with hospital funding for two nurse practitioners. I designed the model after visiting several sites, including Johns Hopkins, Boston University Home Medical Service, the Urban Medical Group in East Boston, the Rochester Home Health Care Team, and St. Vincent's Hospital in New York. The Richmond model is most like Urban Medical but is based at a hospital rather than community health centers and is focused exclusively on home care, like the Rochester team. Our projected load of 60 patients per nurse practitioner came from Urban Medical. When MCV Home Care patients are hospitalized, I often care for them with help from inpatient nurse practitioners who support the faculty practice. Here are some of the lessons I have learned.

Independence

The degree of independence and the process of supervision and physician support for nurse practitioners providing home care differs from other settings, where on-site consultation with physicians and other professionals is usually readily available. At home, medical decisions are more challenging for our nurse practitioners. The medical consequences of incorrect action rest more fully on their shoulders, and these decisions can also place burdens on patients and families. For example, a home care patient was recently found to have a possible perirectal abscess, a condition that may require inpatient surgery. Appropriately, the patient was brought to the emergency room, where she fortunately proved to have only cellulitis (a local skin infection). The decision to transport the patient led to two ambulance rides, several hours in the emergency room, and much cost.

Consider a decision to treat at home. A home care nurse practitioner initially saw a woman who had become difficult for her family to handle because of progressive dementia, probably from Alzheimer's disease. Then we received several calls from home health agency nurses about rapid heart rates. The nurse practitioner visited and found the patient's heart rate markedly elevated at 140, with a slightly reduced blood pressure. Though the woman was slightly more confused than usual, she was physically stable. The home ECG first appeared to indicate only a benign sinus tachycardia, but when the nurse practitioner inserted a bladder catheter to obtain a urine specimen, the heart rate abruptly dropped to normal, suggesting that a more serious supraventricular arrhythmia had occurred. We discussed the likelihood that this demented patient would tear a home heart rhythm monitor to pieces. We also knew she would resist hospital care and might well suffer iatrogenic illness there. After talking with the family, we decided to treat her empirically at home. This was a complex decision based on observations by a nurse practitioner in the field.

Compared to office patients, home care patients have more numerous problems and more frequent changes in medical status. Individual decisions are more complex, and complex situations arise more often. In an office, nurse practitioners may handle 70% of the problems and half of all patients with little or no physician input. In home care, physician input is needed more frequently, including a need to confer from the house on 10% of visits. A home care patient or a caregiver might report chest pain, leg swelling, shortness of breath, arm or leg weakness, abdominal pain, diarrhea, vomiting, fever, rectal bleeding, confusion, falls, or other potentially serious symptoms, most of which can be safely managed at home.

Unlike nurse practitioners in nursing homes, home care practitioners lack a supporting cast of nurses and other professionals. Nursing home patients are under some degree of constant professional observation, which is rarely present at home. This again increases the importance of accurate assessment and decision making. Knowing each of their 60 cases very well, the home care practitioners often intervene medically without consulting. Yet backup from a physician with whom the practitioner has a mutually trusting relationship and who preferably knows the case must be prompt when it is needed. Confirmatory testing at home, including lab work, ECGs, X rays, and even more sophisticated modalities like ultrasound, become more important as acuity increases. It takes longer for nurse practitioners to be comfortable with this level of independence than in roles where consultation is easier.

Acceptance of Nurse Practitioners, or "I Want to See the Doctor"

Unlike office practice, where nurse practitioners are now generally well accepted, the issue of patient, family, and physician comfort with independently functioning home care nurse practitioners has been little studied. Early on, Nelson[45] found that 63% of families felt physician assistants could make the first house call, reporting back to the physician; 15% were opposed, and 22% were unsure. Responses were similar regarding office visits.

Our experience at MCV Home Care is that most families are comfortable with nurse practitioners making management decisions once patients and families understand the nurse practitioners' role and their relationship with our physicians. To facilitate this understanding, we provide an introductory brochure, describing the extra training involved. Nurse practitioners carefully define their role as members of a physician-led team. Some families come to rely heavily on the nurse practitioners and need little physician input. Other families or patients expect frequent direct physician contact. The issues are trust, confidence in the nonphysicians' skills and awareness of their limits, the quality of communication, and underlying societal values, which give physicians final authority.

Defining the frequency for direct physician involvement in a given case is an issue for all teams of physicians and professional care providers, regardless of the setting. An analogy between home care and office teams is appropriate, as medical home care teams are like mobile offices. Most nurse practitioner office visits do not result in direct patient-physician contact. Yet the physician and the office nurse practitioner must decide when and how often the physician should see the patient. One cannot easily define specific guidelines for an ideal mixture of physician and nurse house calls, due to the heterogeneity of the clinical and social situations. The experience of established home care teams may prove the best guide. Ideally, physicians should see home care patients at intervals that make the nurse practitioner, patient, family, and physician comfortable with the process of care. Reflecting this comfort, formal demands for physician consultation should then be infrequent. Physicians should always provide prompt consultation on direct request unless they plan to use the emergency department for backup.

As nurse practitioners and physicians work together, the intervals between physician contacts may lengthen. Similarly, as a new patient's plan of care and the trajectory of the illness(es) become clear, the need for direct physician involvement may lessen. Two-thirds or more of the visits to our seriously ill patients are handled by nurse practitioners. We have satisfied patients who have received more than 90% of their care from nurse practitioners and whose chart reviews and stable course at home testify to high-quality care for many years.

Physicians and nurse practitioners must remain alert to the potential for malpractice litigation. Fortunately, this has been rare in home care for several reasons. However, physicians and nurse practitioners must consider how families would feel and how they might react if patients do poorly.

In some situations, family expectations lead to more urgent physician consultation or referrals to the hospital for acute care rather than treating at home. These can be anxiety-filled moments, particularly for the inexperienced. Malpractice concerns will occasionally cause physicians to make housecalls in support of their nurse practitioners, even though both are comfortable with decisions made by phone.

Generally speaking, physicians support the idea of professional provider house calls. Unpublished data from my 1988 survey of Virginia primary care physicians showed that 92% believed solo house calls by nurse providers would sometimes be helpful. Third-party reimbursement, closely followed by patient acceptance, were important considerations. Unpublished data from our 1990 national survey[1] of internists and family physicians also showed that 22% of 1,161 respondents used alternative providers for solo house calls. Given an acute, nonemergent complaint, 15% of physicians would make a house call, and 3% would send an office nurse, nurse practitioner, or physician assistant. When asked which factors would encourage more house calls by professional care providers, third-party payment and better patient acceptance had approximately equal weight and were far more important than legal risk. Reimbursement commonly was the "single most important" factor. Based on my home care experience, physicians' concern about patient acceptance may derive from inexperience. Most families accept nurse practitioner house calls as long as physicians remain involved.

Personnel Resources, Team Dynamics, and Burnout

Operating a home care practice that joins physicians and other professionals relies on awareness of team dynamics and on maintaining healthy working relationships. This requires frequent team meetings and frank discussions of conflicts. MCV Home Care staff meet weekly for 90 minutes to discuss both patient care and team issues. Home care can be more frustrating and tiring than other types of practice, so team members need room in their schedules for provider respite. This relates to several considerations beyond the complexity of the medical decisions. Home care brings dreary paperwork and care coordination work, which are often neither clinical nor enjoyable. There is much death and dying and much chronic pain. Like oncology and AIDS care, home care can take a toll on the empathetic. And in home care one finds many situations in which there is no satisfactory resolution. When the team finds itself caught between needy patients and a societal system not meeting their needs, having a team social worker can be a great help. Social workers from home health agencies are involved only intermittently due to Medicare regulations, and community-based social workers from public programs like the Public Health Department, Medicaid, or Adult Protective Services may be over-burdened or may have limited roles. Medical home care teams need their own social workers for the benefit of both team members and patients.

There are rewards that counterbalance the stresses. Home care offers an opportunity to address unmet needs and engenders a valued sense of camaraderie and independence. Another factor that has enabled me to attract excellent nurse practitioners to the often arduous work of home care is the opportunity for learning and the challenge offered by the medical complexities. The close connection between our team's physicians and nurse practitioners affords both disciplines the chance to learn from each other and to grow. There is freedom of movement, clinical variety, and diversity of care settings.

Still, the threat of burnout must not be taken lightly. A wise team leader builds flexibility into the schedule and controls the patient census, recognizing that there will be unpredictable peaks and valleys in demand. Peaks are characterized by a series of crises, times of high stress, and consequent staff fatigue. There must also be some lulls when staff reconstitute physical and emotional reserves. If the caseload is too great, there will be inadequate time for recovery, and burnout will surely follow.

This raises the critical issue of personnel resources. Few nurse practitioners or physicians are interested in home care as a major clinical focus. Replacing lost team members can be difficult. Therefore, a future in which medical home care teams are the customary sources of care for most homebound patients would require changes in student selection and post-graduate curricula and reimbursement for nonphysician disciplines. We would need several thousand more providers (see chapter 10). Because of these staffing concerns, the present arrangement, in which chronic home care mostly centers on physician office practices, will persist. If each practice serves 30 to 50 homebound patients per primary care physician, wear-and-tear on home care teams will be lessened and the shortage of future home care specialists will be less acute.

Interfaces with Other Providers

In home care, nurse practitioners often initiate or change orders given to other nurses. Usually, this works well, but occasional problems can arise.

Experienced home health agency nurses sometimes feel that nurse practitioners lack the expertise or medical knowledge to alter the nurses' care plans. In addition, some physician specialists are less accepting of referrals forwarded by nurse practitioners. I introduce our nurse practitioners to my subspecialized colleagues. Over time my need for direct involvement in referrals decreases as the practitioners establish credibility. Still, my active, ongoing interaction with specialist physician colleagues is clearly important. Physicians expect to interact with physicians.

Monitoring Quality of Care

In our office practice, physicians commonly review charts of all patients seen by nurse practitioners. This enhances continuity and is one approach to monitoring quality. Another is periodic, scheduled chart review, which is laborious and cumbersome. Using computerized data to monitor intervals between visits, prescribing patterns, and health maintenance is also effective, assuming that good data management systems exist. Patient satisfaction surveys make another valid approach.

In home care the same principles apply. Team meetings afford one opportunity to focus on care quality. The main strengths and weaknesses of home care teams and individual providers become apparent through frequent contact. Concurrent chart review is difficult because the charts are "in motion." However, with fewer charts to review, periodic scheduled chart review can work in home care; a rotating biannual review is one model we have used. Eventually, computerized medical records may make concurrent review more practical for home care, and I believe this will be the best option. Meanwhile, we use the MCV Home Care database to monitor relationships between emergency room or hospital inpatient care and house calls, the frequency of early hospital readmissions, compliance with pneumonia and influenza vaccination, documentation of patients' terminal care preferences, and other measures of care process. Such administrative research is particularly important to ensure quality when care is provided outside structured settings.

Reimbursement

Payment for professional care provider services in nursing homes and current restrictive policies regarding home care work were reviewed earlier. In chapter 12, I try to define reasonable payment for nurse practitioner housecalls and other home care work. The approximate breakeven figure is about $65 per nurse practitioner house call, assuming an efficient and clinically responsible operation, using full-time nurse practitioners who do a lot of care management. The $65 does not include home care office overhead, which is low. Considering my present situation, where Medicaid pays $32.10, Medicare pays nothing, and most private carriers follow Medicare, changes will be needed if the potential of professional care providers in home care is to be realized. Currently, such providers must operate within a larger system such as a home health agency, a hospital-based home care program, or a capitated risk contract. Private physician offices can't afford the luxury.

FUTURE CHALLENGES

On the important issue of professional care provider independence, which is now defined by state and federal law and by professional licensing organizations, I generally believe that physicians and other care providers should work together in a collaborative, collegial relationship. I do not believe professional care providers should seek fully independent practice status.

This position is opposed by some advocates, whose case is strongly stated by Barbara Safriet in a thorough analysis.[9] Current policies are inconsistent. If these professionals can reliably provide care in under-served areas, why should populous, affluent areas be different? State laws differ in their effects on professionals, and various regulatory boards have variously hindered sensible policies such as the development of prescriptive authority, thereby restricting professionals' practice. There is much inequity. Advocates for independent status argue that full realization of the professional provider role and full respect for professional competency will never be achieved without direct federal reimbursement and authority for independent practice by professional regulatory boards.

I disagree. It appears to me that we are experiencing the growing pains of new professional disciplines coming into a world where powerful, established traditions in medicine and nursing have evolved over centuries. The fact that many nurses and physicians have never worked with professional providers underlies their reluctance to accept the new role. The same is true of the general public, which lacks positive experiences on which to base a changing paradigm. Correcting this problem does not require full independence. Passage of time and broad-based promotion of the professional role will realize the necessary change without creating another class of primary care providers.

Lest I be misunderstood, I am not principally concerned about competition between physicians and professional care providers. Rather, I see patients frequently needing the involvement of physicians whose level of training, knowledge and experience is greater than that of most professional care providers. Although 70% of encounters can be managed independently by nonphysicians, this does not translate to 70% of patients. Periodically and unpredictably, patients develop problems that require physician involvement. Furthermore, most professional care providers do not want a completely independent role. This is particularly true in home care, where multiple serious illnesses often coexist. Rather than having patients followed primarily by professional care providers and referred for physician care when they get sicker, it makes better sense for physicians and professional care providers to work side by side, mutually respectful and collaborative and both familiar with the patients. Then, as complex problems emerge, physicians can respond quickly and appropriately, and the interaction will be smoother.

Differential reimbursement, an inequity that is a sore point for many professional providers, is a separate but related concern. The current basis for professional compensation includes not only the work provided during a service but also the cost of preparing for practice. This premise, which has solid foundations, would oppose simply offering "equal pay for equal work." As we evolve to systems wherein fee-for-service thinking is obsolete, where services are measured by cost and by effectiveness, and where mechanisms for underwriting medical education are changed, the basis for provider compensation will also evolve.

Under capitation the value of providers' work will be determined by regional managers of systems and care teams will be organized to maximize cost-effectiveness. Differential compensation for identical services will be less problematic because we will focus on the total cost of caring for populations rather than the cost of individual services. New provider classes may emerge, including individuals trained specifically for outpatient primary care with little acute care expertise. Acute care may be delivered almost exclusively by "designated hitters." No discipline has fully espoused this radical strategy during professional education, though operationally many providers now find themselves in roles for which much of their education and training has only indirect application.

In the future will we be able to justify the cost of our current educational approach? Perhaps we should radically change direction. We might base our medical care system on a new type of primary care provider, located at a level of training somewhere between the professional care provider and the physician, emphasizing more nursing values than we currently incorporate in physician education. This would require us to change the deeply held societal belief in the healing role of physicians, to change the very concept of the relationship between doctor and patient, and it would be a major cultural transformation. Given the current education of professional care providers, it would also require more extensive education for the new provider class, increasing cost and increasing salaries.

On the other hand, we could alter medical student selection and medical education to produce more primary care physicians, humanistic in their values, holistic in approaching patients, skilled in probabilistic reasoning, and trained to work in close, respectful accord with other disciplines. At the same time, we could enhance and validate the role of professional care providers as members of a team and correspondingly modify their education to prepare for a more independent yet collaborative role. I prefer this vision.

In either case, I wish to strongly endorse the value of professional care providers. This value does not lie primarily where many place it, that is, in absorbing those aspects of health care delivery that are less popular with many physicians: rural care, care of the urban poor, long-term care, psychosocial aspects of physician-patient relationships, primary care, episodic care, and patient teaching. Rather, I welcome the contribution of respected professional colleagues with complementary skills to a team effort directed toward optimizing patient care and meeting the needs of varied populations. This, I hope, will increasingly include home care. We have a long road to travel.

In summary, viewing home care broadly and keeping efficiency in mind, much of the clinical data gathering, analysis, and decision making can be done by a team of nurses, nurse practitioners, therapists, and social workers. Nevertheless, involvement by a physician with home care experience, who is integral to the team and has an accurate understanding of the home situation, is also vital. The next chapter will discuss more fully the guidelines home care physicians should use in defining their roles, in resolving the thorny question of when to make house calls, and in clinically managing their home care practices.

REFERENCES

1. Keenan JM, Boling PA, Schwartzberg JG, Olson L, Schneidermann M, McCaffrey DJ, Ripsin CM. A national survey of the home visiting practice and attitudes of family physicians and internists. *Arch Intern Med.* 1992; 152:2025–2032.
2. Keenan JM, Hepburn KW, Ripsin CM, Webster L, Bland CJ. A survey of Minnesota home care agencies' perceptions of physician behaviors. *Family Medicine.* 1992; 24(2):142–144.
3. Creditor MC. Hazards of hospitalization of the elderly. *Ann Intern Med.* 1993; 118(3):219–223.
4. Boling PA, Keenan JM, Schwartzberg JS, Retchin SM, Olson L, Schneiderman M. Reported home health agency referrals by internists and family physicians. *J Am Geriatr Soc.* 1992; 40:1241–1249.
5. Altemeier TM, Pattee JF, Wagner PN. Core educational objectives for the administrative aspects for medical direction in nursing homes. *Journal of Medical Direction.* 1992; 2(2):59–66.
6. Zimmer JG, Watson NM, Levenson SA. Nursing home medical directors: Ideals and realities. *J Am Geriatr Soc.* 1993; 41:127–130.
7. Elon R. The nursing home medical director role in transition. *J Am Geriatr Soc.* 1993; 41:131–135.
8. Office of Technology Assessment. *Nurse Practitioners, Physician Assistants, and Certified Nurse-Midwives: A Policy Analysis.* Washington, DC: Author; 1986. Health Technology Case Study 37.
9. Safriet BJ. Health care dollars and regulatory sense: The role of advanced practice nursing. *Yale Journal on Regulation.* 1992; 9:417–488.
10. Yankauer A, Sullivan J. The new health professionals: Three examples. *Annu Rev Public Health.* 1982; 3:249–276.
11. Ebersole P. Gerontological nurse practitioners past and present. *Geriatr Nurs.* 1985; July/August:219–222.
12. Salkever DS, Skinner EA, Steinwachs DM, Katz H. Episode-based efficiency comparisons for physicians and nurse practitioners. *Med Care.* 1982; 20(2):143–153.
13. Holmes GC, Livingston G, Bassett RE, Mills E. Nurse clinician productivity using a relative value scale. *Health Serv Res.* 1977; 269–283.
14. Weiner JP, Steinwachs DM, Williamson JW. Nurse practitioner and physician assistant practices in three HMO's: Implications for future US health manpower needs. *J Public Health,* 1986; 76:507–511.
15. Nelson EC, Jacobs AR, Breer PE, Johnson KG. Impact of physician's assistants on patient visits in ambulatory care practices. *Ann Intern Med.* 1975; 82:608–612.

16. Spitzer WO, Sackett DL, Sibley JC, Roberts RS, Gent M, Kergin DJ, Hackett BC, Olynich A. The Burlington Randomized Trial of the Nurse Practitioner. *N Engl J Med.* 1974; 290:251–256.

17. Sackett DL, Spitzer WO, Gent M, Robets RS, et al. The Burlington Randomized Trial of the Nurse Practitioner: Health outcomes of patients. *Ann Intern Med.* 1974; 80:137–142.

18. Nichols LM. Estimating costs of underusing advanced practice nurses. *Nursing Economics.* 1992; 10(5):343–351.

19. Record JC, McCally M, Schweitzer SO, Blomquist RM, Berger BD. New health professions after a decade and a half: Delegation, productivity and costs in primary care. *J Health Politi Policy Law.* 1980; 5:470–497.

20. Regan DM, Harbert KR. Measuring the financial productivity of physician assistants. *Medical Group Management Journal.* 1991; 38(6):46–52.

21. Mendenhall RC, Repicky PA, Neville RE. Assessing the utilization and productivity of nurse practitioners and physician's assistants: Methodology and findings on productivity. *Med Care.* 1980; 18:609–623.

22. Merenstein JH, Wolfe H, Barker KM. The use of nurse practitioners in a general practice. *Med Care.* 1974; 12:445–452.

23. Smith CW. Patient attitudes toward physicians' assistants. *J Fam Pract.* 1981; 13(2):201–204.

24. Zikmund WG, Miller SJ. A factor analysis of attitudes of rural health care consumers toward nurse practitioners. *Research in Nursing and Health.* 1979; 2:85–90.

25. Sox HC. Quality of care by nurse practitioners and physician's assistants: A ten-year perspective. *Ann Intern Med.* 1979; 91:459–468.

26. Weston JL. *Annotated Bibliography of NCHSR Research on Nonphysician Primary Care Providers, 1969–1989.* Rockville, MD: Agency for Health Care Policy and Research, Public Health Service, U.S. Department of Health and Human Services. Report No. AHCPR 90-13 (NCHSR).

27. Ramsay JA, McKenzie JK, Fish DG. Physicians and nurse practitioners: Do they provide equivalent care? *Am J Public Health.* 1982; 72(1):55–57.

28. Maulle WF. Screening for colorectal cancer by nurse endoscopists. *N Engl J Med.* 1994; 330(3):183–187.

29. Slome C, Wetherbee H, Daly M, Christensen K, Meglen M, Thiede H. Effectiveness of certified nurse-midwives. *Am J Obstet Gynecol.* 1974; 124(2):177–182.

30. Graveley EA, Littlefield JH. A cost-effectiveness analysis of three staffing models for the delivery of low-risk prenatal care. *Am J Public Health.* 1992; 82(2):180–184.

31. Runyan JW. The Memphis chronic disease program: Comparisons in outcome and the nurse's extended role. *JAMA.* 1975; 231(3):264–267.

32. Hill F, Bird HA, Harmer R, Wright V, Lawton C. An evaluation of the effec-

tiveness, safety and acceptability of a nurse practitioner in a rheumatology outpatient clinic. *Br J Rheumatol.* 1994; 33:283–288.

33. Dutters MJ, Harlan WR. Evaluation of physician assistants in rural primary care. *Arch Intern Med.* 1978; 138:224–228.

34. Kane RL, Garrard J, Skay CL, Radosevich DM, Buchanan JL, McDermott SM, Arnold SB, Kepferle L. Effects of a geriatric nurse practitioner on process and outcome of nursing home care. *Am J Public Health.* 1989; 79:1271–1277.

35. Garrard J, Kane RL, Radosevich DM, Skay CL, Arnold SB, Kepferle L, McDermott SM, Buchanan JL. Impact of geriatric nurse practitioners on nursing-home residents' functional status, satisfaction, and discharge outcomes. *Med Care.* 1990; 28(3):271–283.

36. Kane RA, Kane RL, Arnold S, Garrard J, McDermott S, Kepferle L. Geriatric nurse practitioners as nursing home employees: Implementing the role. *Gerontologist.* 1988; 28(4):469–477.

37. Buchanan JL, Bell RM, Arnold SB, Wistberger C, Kane RL, Garrard J. Assessing cost effects of nursing-home-based geriatric nurse practitioners. *Health Care Financing Administration Review.* 1990; 11(3):67–78.

38. Kane RL, Garrard J, Buchanan JL, Rosenfeld A, Skay C, McDermott S. Improving primary care in nursing homes. *J Am Geriatr Soc.* 1991; 39:359–367.

39. Master RJ, Feltin M, Jainchill J, Mark R, Kavesh WN, Rabkin MT, Turner B, Bachrach S, Lennox S. A continuum of care for the inner city: Assessment of its benefits for Boston's elderly and high-risk populations. *N Engl J Med.* 1980; 302;1434–1440.

40. Kolassa J, Katz PR, Karuza J. Report from the AMA Professional Activities Census: Extent and profile of nursing home practice. *J Am Geriatr Soc.* 1994; 42(11):SA72. Abstract.

41. Ginsburg PB, LeRoy LB et al., eds. Physician Payment Review Commission. Medicaid Payment Policies for Nonphysician Practitioner Services. In *Annual Report to Congress of the Physician Payment Review Commission.* Washington, DC: Author; 1993; chap. 16.

42. Kavesh W, Bachrach S. Nursing home innovation in the public arena. *Journal of Aging and Social Policy.* 1990; 2(2):87–106.

43. Stuck AE, Aronow HV, Seiner A, et al. A trial of annual in-home comprehensive geriatric assessments for elderly people living in the community. *N Engl J Med.* 1995; 333:1184–1189.

44. Della Penna RD. A model long term care program using geriatricians and geriatric nurse practitioners in an HMO. Presented at the annual meeting of the American Geriatrics Society. May 19, 1994; Los Angeles, Calif.

45. Nelson EC, Jacobs AR, Johnson KG. Patients' acceptance of physician's assistants. *JAMA.* 1974; 228:63–67.

CHAPTER 4

Home Health Care Practice Guidelines for Physicians

I n 1987 the American Medical Association (AMA) convened an expert panel to develop home care guidelines for physicians. The panel had 14 physicians and 1 nurse, including high-tech home care specialists, primary care physicians, home health agency medical directors, academic physicians, and private practitioners. By November 1990, after several meetings, the group reached consensus. Then in 1992, capping a process of critical editing and revision, the AMA published *Guidelines for the Medical Management of the Home Care Patient,* a useful $3 monograph. This chapter explores the clinical aspects of two related domains of home care practice: house calls and home care management.

HOUSE CALLS: WHY, WHEN, AND HOW OFTEN?

One hotly debated issue was defining reasonable expectations for house calls and for other direct contact between physicians and patients who are homebound or who receive physician-ordered home care. This was the result.

For some relatively functional patients, home care needs may be adequately defined in an office setting. However, for most patients, in-home assessments are preferable and may even be critical. In-home assessments can be highly efficient ways to save time in diagnosis, medical decision making, and communication among all team members. These assessments may be performed by physicians or by other health professionals who are in close communication with the physician, depending on the circumstances. The timing and frequency of assessment and reassessment will vary. The following are general guidelines:

Physicians should know the status of their patients. The number of home visits by the physician or others should meet the requirement that the physician knows the patient's current status.

Patients with complex, deteriorating, or fluctuating conditions require more frequent visits. The number should be at least comparable to the visit frequency required to manage that condition in another setting. (AMA *Guidelines,* p. 9)

The group recognized that arbitrary criteria for house calls would be neither practical nor consistent with good medical practice, where care is adjusted to need. The homebound are heterogeneous, so their needs vary. Yet the statement means that home care patients should be followed as closely as their conditions warrant, even if this poses a challenge for physicians who are balancing multiple priorities.

How often should physicians visit homebound patients? Examples may help. GW is a 70-year-old woman who had extensive surgery for vulvar cancer, then repair of an iliac artery aneurysm. She was left with a massively swollen leg and a large open groin wound. She was bedfast at home for a year, then slowly started to walk, to use a seat-lift chair, and to resume normal activities. Her niece is a nurse who reliably calls if problems arise. I visit GW on demand, once or twice a year.

EA was my patient, a 70-year-old woman with polycythemia vera (an indolent type of leukemia) that caused clotting of many arteries, amputation of both legs, and heart failure. She too had extensive repair for a large iliac pseudoaneurysm after a limb salvage procedure. EA then lived on her couch in a housing project apartment with no phone. She was obstinate, and she was inconsistent about taking medicine. Her daughter, volatile and medically naïve, was not a reliable source of information. EA often "sent for me" when she was very sick, but if I didn't take the initiative to visit her every few months, she often ended up in the hospital, with cardiac problems.

Thus, house call frequency is dictated by the need to know patients well enough to make sound medical decisions and also for patients and families to know and trust physicians so that therapy will proceed smoothly when problems arise. House call frequency also depends on the quality of the reports by other home health care team members, such as nurses or family members, as discussed in the preceding chapter.

National population-wide estimates are that physicians average one or two house calls annually per chronically homebound patient (see chapter 9). These patients may receive additional physician care in offices, emergency rooms, or hospitals, but the burden associated with access is high, and outpatient physician contacts are far less frequent than is standard for other similar populations. For example, physician or professional care provider examination of nursing home patients is federally mandated within 48 hours of admission, monthly for 90 days, and every 60 days thereafter, with extra visits if needed. As outpatients, ambulatory elders in poor health average 10 or 12 physician office visits a year.[1] We might debate these standards, but the discrepancy between these two reference groups and the homebound is so large that the unmet need of the homebound is indisputable.

One concern is the lack of hard data proving that house calls are worthwhile, despite the anecdotal support that abounds in the practices of physicians who regularly make house calls. There is no doubt that one gains new information.[2] After a comprehensive clinic-based evaluation by an experienced geriatric assessment team, house calls to the same patients identified 1.7 new problems on average. These included safety issues plus assorted medical and functional needs (see Table 4.1).

Discovering unreported needs during house calls is not news. In 1972, Williamson found previously unrecognized disabilities, mobility impairment, sensory deficits, and assorted medical and neuropsychiatric problems.[3] Ramsdell's study is unique for first completing a clinic-based evaluation. Perhaps rightly, many physicians might consider that some of the less "medical" problems found by Ramsdell's group would best be addressed by other professional care providers, as they are in Texas[4] and at UCLA.[5] In the latter case, 4.9 new problems were found among patients receiving regular care from private physicians. The needs found by Ramsdell's group were often medical: gait and balance disorders (24%), cardiac problems (7%), neoplasm (4%), and depression (8%). They advised the types of interventions shown in Table 4.2.

Ramsdell's group made a one-time assessment. In my longitudinal home care practice, I think that we find proportionately more new med-

TABLE 4.1 Problems Newly Diagnosed by Home Visit

Category	No. (%) problems
Safety	55 (22)
Psychobehavioral	59 (23)
Family/stress	52 (20)
Nutrition	24 (9)
Activities of daily living	12 (5)
Financial	7 (3)
Medical	46 (18)

From "The Yield of a Home Visit in the Assessment of Geriatric Patients," by Ramsdell et al., 1989, *Journal of the American Geriatrics Society, 37*, 17–24. Copyright © 1989 Williams & Wilkins. Reprinted with permission.

TABLE 4.2 Recommendations Newly Made After Home Visit

Category	No. (%) recommendations
Safety measures	126 (31)
Social interventions (e.g., day care)	52 (13)
General health	33 (8)
Nutrition	28 (7)
Medication changes	14 (3)
Home care services	25 (6)
Caregiver support/education	81 (20)
Preventive health	27 (7)
Institutional placement	24 (6)

From "The Yield of a Home Visit in the Assessment of Geriatric Patients," by Ramsdell et al., 1989, *Journal of the American Geriatrics Society, 37*, 17–24. Copyright © 1989 Williams & Wilkins. Reprinted with permission.

ical problems because medical conditions change faster than social support systems do. Social supports are often greatly stressed, but their inherent stability is a basic premise for home care, whereas deteriorating health, inherently unstable, is what makes people homebound.

Patient choice may also affect house call frequency. In a study comparing ambulatory elders with middle-aged adults, the elders sought care sooner after the onset of symptoms.[6] However, because they may attribute symptoms to old age, or because they must consider cost, immobility, or other factors, some older patients don't seek medical attention despite needing help.[7] For those with severe functional impairment, good support systems increase the frequency of physician contacts, and economic deprivation is a negative factor.[8] Delays can have serious consequences, which may be forestalled by timely, judicious intervention. EA was such a case.

Because of technical research issues (see chapter 6), it is difficult to convincingly connect physicians' increased involvement and awareness of problems to improved outcomes or lower cost. For now, I posit the inherent value of having better information about patients. Consider a patient whose mantel holds 15 pill bottles, some long outdated. These include three bottles of digoxin, two of which are labeled "Digoxin" and one labeled "Lanoxin." The patient takes a pill from each bottle every day, making a dangerous overdose. Consider the malnourished patient whose refrigerator contains only a few pigs' feet, some dried-out bacon, and an uncovered bowl of partially eaten potatoes. See the half-full liquor bottle and the empty pill bottle beside the chair of a half-blind, chair-bound man with kidney failure whose lab tests always show acidosis despite many prescriptions for bicarbonate. He steadfastly denies drinking and swears he takes the medicine. Later, dialysis is being discussed, which requires compliance between treatments. The physician, having made this visit, is now ready to authoritatively discuss the home situation with the nephrologist when this major decision is made.

At the risk of tedium, here are other examples. These are the daily bread of home care physicians. One may find a totally dependent patient repeatedly left unattended by a caregiver who reports no trouble meeting caregiving responsibilities, and only then may the physician understand why the bedsores (pressure ulcers) do not heal. Or notice the loose, ventilation grate, a virtual trapdoor in the hallway floor between the room of a blind, unsteady old woman and her second-floor bathroom. Observe plastic carpet covers laid by the bed of a frail, chronically incontinent woman and watch her stocking-clad feet slide from under her as she tries to reach her commode—a hip fracture in the offing. Watch the severely arthritic patient struggle to rise from her comfortable chair and grab a walker someone prescribed at hospital discharge, and know that without physical therapy, institutionalization is imminent. Experience the oppressive summer heat in a room where a diabetic stroke patient who swallows liquids with difficulty spends her dehydrated days, and then know the need to press for an air conditioner.

Often these problems can and should be discovered by other professionals and communicated to the physician. However, there is truth in the saying about a picture being worth a thousand words. The perspective gained by entering a home cannot be effectively conveyed by verbal or written descriptions. There is also a continuous clinical reasoning process during physician-patient encounters, an integration of observations, pathophysiology, and therapy—concurrent discovery of new problems and the making of additional relevant observations as the session proceeds. Imagine asking physicians in any other context to make serious medical judgments from a distance, without actually seeing the patients.

Video images may become one useful adjunct, particularly if we can solve the problems of confidentiality and patient comfort with video records of their homes. However, with due respect to video technology, entering the home still gives an irreplaceable sense of the place. The physician who has been to a home, even infrequently, knows things about that patient's situation that no other physician can know. Moreover, beyond information gathering and problem solving, a special relationship is engendered by the house call. The physician's presence conveys, perhaps better than any words or personal mannerisms, the physician's commitment. If the physician assumes a respectful approach as a guest in the home, a powerful bond usually forms quickly. Not only does the physician care enough to use some of a busy schedule for this activity, but caregiver and patient are both relieved of the burden imposed by traveling to see the physician.

Finally, the truly unique contribution of home visiting by physicians and professional care providers lies in the ability to immediately follow assessments with treatment. Interventions may involve acute problems like heart failure, infection, and stroke or chronic problems like hypertension and incontinence. Taken all together, the reasons given above make a powerful generic argument for house calls.

WHEN IS A HOUSE CALL INDICATED?

Several surveys bear on this question, beginning with a 1972 paper that eloquently defines many key issues.[9] Surveyors usually ask physicians about indications for house calls in their actual practices, which is differ-

TABLE 4.3 Reasons for Making House Calls

| | Percentage responding sometimes/often | | |
Reason for house call	Family medicine	Internal medicine	General pediatrics
Acute illness	53	42	56
Chronic illness	80	84	42
Terminal care	86	81	34
Evaluate home/family situation	18	18	21
Emotional problem/family crisis	16	16	20
Emotional support to patient/family	27	23	33
Death pronouncement	39	33	11

From "House Call Practices: A Comparison by Specialty," by Adelman, Fredman, & Knight *Journal of Family Practice, 39.* 1, 39–44; 1994 used by permission of Appleton & Lang, Inc.

ent from asking what they would recommend in an ideal world, but the answers show the priorities. Adelman's 1991 survey of family physicians, general internists, and pediatricians found the results shown in Table 4.3.[10]

Among principal reasons for house calls to adults, providers listed cancer (73%), stroke (56%), heart failure (47%), dementia (39%), paraplegia/quadriplegia (40%), pressure ulcers (27%), arthritis (27%), mechanical ventilation (9%), and AIDS (7%). Pediatricians reported newborn care (41%) and cancer (18%) as their usual indications. Adelman's results are very similar to data from the 1990 national survey of internists and family physicians who ranked the strength of indications for house calls,[11] though there were some differences in the phrasing of items (see Table 4.4).

In 1987, Utah physicians rated factors influencing decisions about making a house call from 5 (very important) to 0 (unimportant).[12] By far the strongest indication involved access. Being bedbound or housebound rated 4.75, followed by being elderly (3.73) and recent disability (3.73), and events such as heart attack, stroke, or trauma. Similar lists have been recorded by others.[13,14] And Warburton's 1976 survey of 290 family physicians found that 1.3 of 6 weekly house calls were emergency visits.[15] In years past even urgent nocturnal visits were part of U.S. physician practices.[16] The themes are clear. The strongest motivations for house calls are terminal care and patient lack of access to medical care due to immobil-

TABLE 4.4 Reasons for House Calls

	Percentage choosing often/always	
Reason for house call	Internal medicine	Family practice
Assess acute problem	45	26
Manage chronic problems	32	21
Provide terminal care	55	29
Assess home situation	28	14
Pressure from family	61	32
Patient could not afford van/ambulance	54	33
Transportation available but travel too difficult for the patient	57	36
Patient is a long-term patient of the doctor	63	43
To allow the patient to stay at home	48	31
Improve patient compliance	17	15
Postsurgical care	13	11

From "A National Survey of the Home Visiting Practice & Attitudes of Family Physicians & Internists," by Keenan et al., 1992, *Archives of Internal Medicine, 152*, 2025–2032. Copyright © 1992, American Medical Association. Reproduced with permission.

ity from chronic illness, followed by acute care. Psychosocial issues, home assessment, and technical services are important but are less often the driving forces.

Another factor fostering house calls is family pressure. The more actively a physician participates in home care, the more families rely on the physician. This is appropriate and is typical of physician-patient relationships. It is also important for physicians to support family caregivers (see chapter 6). Yet in home care, physician stress rises with the urgency of family requests. The strain increases proportionately to patients' or caregivers' fears, the degree of social and medical instability, and the degree to which people harbor unrealistic expectations. This physician burden is hard to measure, but it is substantial.

The studies noted above suggest a taxonomy of home care problems that indicates need for a physician's personal attention in the home. The more important of these follow.

FACTORS INDICATING NEED FOR A HOUSE CALL

Access

Access problems include lack of available, affordable transportation; the burden on sick patients caused by any mode of transportation; and the imposition on caregivers, who have to leave work, hire baby-sitters, or bring young children along when accompanying homebound patients to see physicians. Considered broadly, these societal costs and burdens may outweigh the cost of house calls.

In part, the access problem follows the gradual development of incompatibility between frail persons and their dwellings. Life's course can make impediments of features once treasured. For instance, in Pittsburgh's Greenfield district, homes are on steep hills, and have many front steps. The steps, a place for social gatherings in youth and middle age, may become a barrier to seeking medical care, although basic needs like nutrition are still well met. Someone must carry the person down the steps. This implies multiple strong porters, physical risk to the porters, legal risk to their employer, and considerable cost. Should these frail people move to life-care communities or rest homes where their needs can be more easily met? Such questions test our basic values.

Access is also influenced by local characteristics like topography, population density, affluence or poverty, and ethnicity while the core issue of frailty remains constant. For example, consider aging Floridians who retired to beachside condos, then lost their independence. Contrast this with a rural town in West Virginia where the elderly stayed behind while the younger generation left, seeking better jobs when the coal and lumber industries weakened. The tide went out and left some of these older people clinging doggedly, like barnacles.

The access problem can be clarified further by dividing the homebound into two groups: those who can't go and those who won't go.[17] The first group has physical problems. The second group includes patients with primary diagnoses of dementia and chronic psychiatric illness. These people, a subset of those with psychiatric illness, most of whom can attend clinics, have a serious access problem.[18]

TABLE 4.5 Selected Diagnoses 1994 MCV Home Care Patients ($N = 651$)

Diagnosis	Number	Diagnosis	Number
Hypertension	295	Gout	29
Stroke	226	Deep vein thrombosis	26
Diabetes mellitus	181	Femur (hip) fracture	25
Congestive heart failure	178	Rheumatoid arthritis	19
Dementia (Not otherwise specified)	151	Breast cancer	15
Alzheimer's disease (probable)	67	Pulmonary embolism	15
Degenerative arthritis	153	Lung cancer	13
Urinary incontinence	149	Mitral valve disease	12
Coronary artery disease	109	Prostate cancer	11
Pressure (decubitus) ulcers	98	Cirrhosis	10
Chronic obst. pulmonary disease	83	Pernicious anemia	9
Anemia (Hgb. <10)	74	Amyotrophic lateral sclerosis	5
Atrial fibrillation	72	Paget's disease (bone)	3
Peripheral arterial disease	70	Pancytopenia	2
Chronic renal failure (creat. ≥2)	60	Hypopituitarism	2
Seizures	54	Leukemia	2
Legal blindness	53	Chronic active hepatitis	1
Recurrent urinary tract infection	46	Addison's disease	1
Depression	38	Uveitis	1

Medical Problems

After access, the second major category indicating a house call is medical need. On one level this is simple: patients are sick and need to see medical providers. These house calls can be grouped: preventive care, diagnostic care, therapeutic care, rehabilitative care, and long-term maintenance care.[19] Alternatively, medical indications can be grouped by diagnosis, as in some of the several studies cited above. The Medical College of Virginia (MCV)Home Care Program database adds the esoteric to the list of common problems found in published physician surveys. At the time of referral, we record all active diagnoses and risk factors, such as osteoporosis. The database has over 300 diagnoses, averaging 5.6 active diagnoses per patient. Selected examples are shown in Table 4.5, and there is a point to listing the esoteric ones.

House calls keep physicians on their toes. Scattered among the common conditions prompting house calls is surprising variety. A patient develops new fluid-filled skin blisters. These might represent excessive fluid pressure in the legs, induced by heart failure or weak leg veins, or infections by yeast (candida), or herpes viruses (shingles). Several patients have developed bullous pemphigoid, a treatable blistering condition distinguished by clinical exam or skin biopsy, easily done at home, from less common but more serious skin conditions that are treated differently. When someone calls about new skin blisters, a well-informed medical provider should see the patient. Likewise, nausea and poor eating may represent medication side effects, worsened kidney failure, a bladder infection, a painless duodenal ulcer caused by arthritis medication, depression, constipation, or something else entirely. The long list of possible home care medical scenarios virtually defies cataloging. Solid medical diagnosis and treatment skills are essential.

Chronic Care and Terminal Care

I consider these to be a spectrum. In reviewing community-based care, Weissert and Cready called the Rochester Home Care Team a "hospice program," reflecting the 30% death rate. The MCV Home Care experience is similar: 21% of 645 patients died within 6 months, and 31% died by 1 year. Average survival is 15 months. Even though we do not selectively enroll "terminal" patients and few have active cancer diagnoses at entry, this is not surprising. Rather, becoming homebound usually marks declining health, creating the strong association between activities of daily living (ADL) deficits and mortality.[20, 21] Yet home care physicians can't afford to be fatalistic. In 1982, Manton showed improvement 2 years later in 15% or 20% of persons with severe functional impairment.

Home care physicians regularly help patients with severe chronic illnesses to cope for an unpredictable length of time. A few will improve. For the rest, unless they die suddenly at home or develop an acute illness and die quickly in the hospital, home care physicians will eventually find themselves helping with terminal care.

Nonmedical Reasons for House Calls

After access to medical care and specific medical problems, we find such needs as gathering information about the home and supporting caregivers. Physician surveys downplay these indications, but the importance of physicians to caregivers must not be underestimated (see chapter 5).

Additionally, i _____ physicians to have personal awareness of the hor _____ dly, physicians are often less adept at evaluating s _____ ne health nurses, social workers, and other case i _____ nderstandings sometimes develop between these p.u.c.ssionals and family caregivers that are related to lack of familiarity with medical issues, and these misunderstandings can occasionally have dramatic, undesirable effects. Physicians can defuse such situations by bringing medical insights into discussions of largely social issues.

Urgent House Calls

Knight notes that most house calls can be made on a routine basis,[22] offers a decision tree to assist with house call decisions, and gives an acronym, "INHOME," that stresses six elements of assessment during house calls: immobility, nutrition, housing, other people, medications, and examination. However, like Warburton's family physicians, we find that in 1996 about 20% of MCV Home Care house calls are still prompted by acute complaints. It takes experience to decide whether a house call is urgently needed. In office practice, if a physician is uncomfortable about offering telephone advice after talking with a patient, the safest option is for the patient to visit the office. Unless the physician makes house calls, the safest option in home care usually involves an emergency room visit. Knowing the patient and knowing home care makes a physician better able to make home care triage decisions wisely.

Contraindications to House Calls and Provider Safety

Just as there are reasons to make house calls, there are reasons not to make house calls. House calls for patient convenience when the patient is fully ambulatory might exemplify such extravagances. Another reason to decline house calls is when professional providers are at personal risk. Physicians not used to home care may suffer misperceptions about risk, based on sociodemographic characteristics of neighborhoods. This is common in Richmond, where in some neighborhoods domestic and drug-related violence are common at night but rare during the day. Accurate assessment of personal risk is important to allow service where service is needed, and to avoid harm. Some recommendations are shown in Figure 4.1.[23]

Recognize potential risk factor and danger signs
- Location of home in a high-crime area
- Race or sex differences between provider and household
- Intoxicated patient/caregiver exhibiting aggressive behavior
- Presence of people who may be criminals

Interventions
- Visit dangerous areas early in the day
- Do not visit dangerous areas after dark
- Call ahead (household can determine if environment is safe)
- Use alternate provider (male in place of female)
- Do not carry medicines and advertise that policy
- Visit in groups of two or more when in very dangerous areas
- Communicate with other professionals regarding unsafe homes
- Give patient alternative sources for care if safety reasons force withdrawal
- Report unsafe homes to agencies for adult protective services

Figure 4.1 Providers' safety during home visits.

CLINICAL PRACTICE GUIDELINES

Given the broad spectrum of indications for house calls, some specific practice guidelines are needed. The AMA guidelines offer a conceptual framework but do not give details about the clinical process of assessment and monitoring. Here we might borrow from recommendations for "Physician Evaluation and Management of Nursing Home Patients,"[24] which readers should consult for helpful details.

ANNUAL EVALUATIONS

Complete annual evaluations in home care have recently been shown to be cost-effective.[25] And in one chronically ill ambulatory group (age ≥ 55) examination 1 year after a previous complete exam turned up one new diagnosis per patient. Some were significant, such as cancer, aortic aneurysm, atrial fibrillation, hypothyroidism, and diabetes, and most responded to therapy.[26]

Laboratory testing in home care is important, given a medically ill population who take many medications. MCV Home Care staff use the diagnostic lab on more than half of urgent visits and 30% of all visits. One study of routine annual laboratory testing in nursing home patients showed that 17% of tests were abnormal and a third of the findings were new.[27] Potential benefits accrued to 17%; and major benefits, to 3%. Thus, there may be reasons for frequent, selective testing in home care. The subject warrants formal study, particularly because new portable technologies, now becoming available, will make feasible a wide variety of on-site tests.

Obviously, each patient's evaluation should be appropriate to individual needs. For example, a severely demented, bedfast patient with poor dentition, fed through a gastrostomy because of dysphagia, may not need comprehensive dental care. Skin care and caregiver needs might be a better focus.

PREVENTIVE CARE

Mammography can also be used selectively: an 87-year-old homebound woman with a benign breast exam, who is dying of heart disease, won't benefit from screening mammography, which also entails a trip to the radiologist. Similar analyses apply to screening for colon, prostate, and uterine cancer. It is easy to follow guidelines for breast and rectal examinations, difficult to do pelvic exams, and burdensome to arrange flexible sigmoidoscopy. However, for some homebound patients, like young women with long life expectancies, screening exams remain important and are too easily overlooked. Cholesterol is another risk factor reasonably disregarded in very frail elders, whereas other preventive measures, such as influenza and pneumococcal vaccination, are very important. At MCV Home Care, we wage a successful vaccination campaign each October, using our database to list patients needing the vaccines and building vaccinations into the visit schedule. Much of the preventive work in home care is also relatively nonmedical: avoiding accidental injury, delaying functional decline, and forestalling provider burnout. In this way home care is relatively unique.

INDICATIONS FOR HOME HEALTH AGENCY AND EQUIPMENT REFERRALS

In chapter 3 we saw that often the largest part of a home care physician's role is being part of an extended interdisciplinary team and recommending or endorsing home care intervention without making house calls. This first requires that the physician recognize situations where home care is needed and is likely to be beneficial. Not all home care patients are chronically homebound, nor are they all afflicted with severe functional impairment. Once the need is known, the next step is to take appropriate action, whether by requesting home health agency care; ordering a cane, a walker, or wheelchair; or simply advising the patient to clear the path between bed and bath, improve lighting, and install bath rails. Here the physician often relies for guidance on the eyes and ears of other home health care professionals, family members, and neighbors.

Clinical indications for referrals to home health agencies overlap with those for house calls. Many diagnoses for which physicians consider house calls mirror the diagnoses that drive agency referrals. The diagnosis related groups (DRGs) for stroke, heart failure, diabetes, chronic lung disease, and renal failure prompted posthospital home care in 15% of cases or more in 1985. On the other hand, surgical DRGs, like those for peripheral arterial disease and major orthopedic procedures, also spur home health care, but these diagnoses are less common indications for house calls, even though many house call patients have these disorders. House calls are primarily made by medical or cognitive service providers, rather than by procedurists.

Internists and family physicians in the 1990 national home care survey were asked about their indications for home health agency referrals.[28] Many were broadly endorsed. Those selected less often included physician's personal satisfaction with home care referrals, management of bedridden pregnancy complications, and assessment of acute medical problems, perhaps reflecting lack of experience and comfort with home care.

Physicians were more comfortable with home health agency care in chronic care situations and terminal illness than in acute illness. Also, overall, physicians were more enthusiastic about home health agency referrals about house calls. Physicians agreed that most patients and families could be taught to perform care at home (over 90%), and that physicians should use home care agencies more (85%). Agreement dropped to near 70% with expression of the attitude that "the home environment and family supports are usually adequate to allow care to be provided at home." Still fewer (about 45%) agreed that "most patients and/or families can be taught to provide complex care activities in the home, including home intravenous therapy." Physicians appeared willing to use more home care, but they became cautious as care became more technical. Active substitution of nursing care for physician house calls was also endorsed. Seventy percent of those not making house calls agreed that "with readily available visiting registered nurses and nursing aides, most home visits by physicians are unnecessary," along with 48% of those making house calls.

Perhaps it would be well to end the discussion of home health agency referrals with thoughts about physician education. Thirty percent of physicians in the 1990 national survey felt they lacked "sufficient knowledge about available community services to personally plan and deliver home health care." In 1989, Minnesota home care agencies agreed.[29]

This is relevant. There are times when physicians could use home health care effectively, yet fail to do so. The need to refer for postoperative wound care or for rehabilitative care after a stroke or joint replacement is well-appreciated. Most physicians are aware of high-tech options like home intravenous therapy. However, consider outpatient referral for a short course of home physical therapy to an arthritic patient who has become deconditioned and is falling or for preoperative home assessment of orthopedic surgery patients. Many physicians do not know that, along with nursing care, physical therapy qualifies for starting Medicare skilled home care. Other patients stay in the hospital for an extra day to make sure their lab results are not changing. Serious physician issues deter such referrals, including paperwork hassles, compensation, and logistical difficulties when initiating and directing home health care, but one of the main problems is that home care does not come to mind quickly enough.

A FINAL WORD ON HOME CARE PHYSICIANS AND HOUSE CALLS

Closing this section, I borrow from a "Letter from New Ollerton." Here a British general practitioner describes a contemporary overseas practice where five generalist physicians care for 10,000 persons living in and around a mining village.[30] This ratio of patients to primary care physicians would be typical for the United States. House calls were made at morning's end based on requests placed with the receptionist. The physician on call for the weekend often made 15 or 20 house calls. The author reported 1,624 visits in 2 years, half requested by patients. Thirty-five percent were planned by the physician for chronic care. In all, 180 visits were made to people who were dying; one patient received 31 visits during her final 9 weeks of life. There were 178 night visits divided among five physicians. An additional fee was attached for night visits, whereas daytime visits were covered by the national health benefit. Dr. Loudon good-humoredly acknowledged other aspects familiar to home care physicians, including missing light bulbs and uncooperative pets. He closed with a reference to Hippocrates (whose famous oath includes the words, "into whatsoever house I shall enter") and a nod to another important home care skill, "the getaway." Somehow, this description seemed about right.

REFERENCES

1. Cunningham P, Cornelius L. *The Medical Expenditure Survey. Use of Health Care: Findings from the SAIAN and Household Survey.* Rockville, MD: Public Health Service, Agency for Health Care Policy and Research; 1993. AHCPR Pub No. 93–0041.
2. Ramsdell JW, Swart JA, Jackson E, Renvall M. The yield of a home visit in the assessment of geriatric patients. *J Am Geriatr Soc.* 1989; 37(1):17–24.
3. Williamson J, Stokoe IH, Gray S, Fisher M, Smith A, McGhee A, Stephenson E. Old people at home: Their unreported needs. *Lancet.* 1964; 1:1117–1120.
4. DeLoach J, Ware T, Knebl J, Weaver J. In-home and needs assessment in homebound low-income black elderly: Second year experience. *J Am Geriatr Soc.* 1994; 42(11):SA70.
5. Fabacher D, Pietruszka F, Josephson K, Linderborn K, Morley JE, Rubenstein LZ. Findings from an In-home assessment. Abstract P136. *J Am Geriatr Soc.* October 1994:SA53; 1994.
6. Leventhal EA, Leventhal H, Schaefer P, Easterling D. Conservation of energy, uncertainty reduction, and swift utilization of medical care among the elderly. *J Gerontol.* 1993; 48(2):P78–P86.
7. Branch LG, Nemeth KT. When elders fail to visit physicians. *Med Care.* 1985; 23:1265–1275.
8. Arling G. Interaction effects in a multivariate model of physician visits by older people. *Med Care.* 1985; 23:361–371.
9. Wickware DS. Three of four family doctors make house calls. *Patient Care.* 1972; 105–118.
10. Adelman AM, Fredman L, Knight AL. House call practices: A comparison by specialty. *J Fam Pract.* 1994; 39:39–44.
11. Keenan JM, Boling PA, Schwartzberg JG, Olson L, Schneidermann M, McCaffrey DJ, Ripsin CM. A national survey of the home visiting practice and attitudes of family physicians and internists. *Arch Intern Med.* 1992; 152:2025–2032.
12. Schueler MS, Harris DL, Goodenough GK, Collette L. House calls in Utah.

West J Med. 1987; 147(1):92–94.

13. Siwek J. House calls: Current status and rationale. *Am Fam Physician.* 1985; 31(4):169–174.

14. Cauthen DB. The house call in current medical practice. *J Fam Pract.* 1981; 13:209–213.

15. Warburton SW, Sadler GR, Eikenberry EF. House call patterns of New Jersey family physicians. *J Fam Pract.* 1977; 4:933–938.

16. Elford RW, Brown JW, Robertson LS, Alpert JJ, Kosa J. A study of house-calls in the practices of general practitioners. *Med Care.* 1972; 10(2):173–178.

17. Wald-Cagan P, Fox A. Characteristics of an elderly population: The can't go vs. the won't go. *Gerontologist.* 1991; 31(5, special issue 2):115.

18. Moscovice I, Lurie N, Christianson J, Finch M, Popkin M, Akhtar MR. Access and use of health services by chronically mentally ill Medicaid beneficiaries. *Health Care Financing Review.* 1993; 14(4):75–87.

19. The Council on Scientific Affairs of the American Medical Association. Home care in the 1990's. *JAMA.* 1990; 263:1241–1244.

20. Wolinsky FD, Callahan CM, Fitzgerald JF, Johnson RJ. Changes in functional status and the risks of subsequent nursing home placement and death. *J Gerontol.* 1993; 48(3):S93–S101.

21. Manton KG. A longitudinal study of functional change and mortality in the United States. *J Gerontol.* 1988; 43(5):S153–S161.

22. Knight AL, Adelman AM. The family physician and home care. *Am Fam Physician.* 1991; 44:1733–1737.

23. Boling PA. Safety in the Home. Chapter 18, pp.159–165. In Yoshikawa TT, Cobbs EL, Brummel-Smith K, eds.: *Ambulatory Geriatric Care,* St. Louis, MO: Mosby-Year Book. Inc; 1993.

24. Ouslander JG, Osterweil D. Physician evaluation and management of nursing home patients. *Ann Intern Med.* 1994; 120:584–592.

25. Stuck AE, Aronow HU, Steiner A, Alessi CA, Bula CJ, Gold MN et al. A trial of annual in-home comprehensive geriatric assessments for elderly people living in the community. *N Engl J Med.* 1995; 333:1184–1189.

26. Moore S, Hamdy RC. The value of an annual physical examination. *J Am Geriatr Soc.* 1992; 40(10):SA69. Abstract.

27. Levinstein MR, Ouslander JG, Rubenstein LZ, Forsythe SB. Yield of routine annual laboratory tests in a skilled nursing home population. *JAMA.* 1987; 258:1909–1915.

28. Boling PA, Keenan JM, Schwartzberg JS, Retchin SM, Olson L, Schneiderman M. Reported home health agency referrals by internists and family physicians. *J Am Geriatr Soc.* 1992; 40:1241–1249.

29. Keenan JM, Hepburn KW, Ripsin CM, Webster L, Bland CJ. A survey of Minnesota home care agencies' perceptions of physician behaviors. *Fam Med.* 1992; 24(2):142–144.

30. Loudon MF. Visiting patients in their homes. *JAMA.* 1988; 260:501–502.

CHAPTER 5

Physicians and Nonmedical Caregivers

N No one disputes that nonmedical caregivers are critical to home care. Furthermore, as our society ages, the number of care recipients will grow, the number of available caregivers will proportionately lessen, and support for caregivers will become increasingly vital. Weissert writes:[1]

> As a society we do little or nothing to relieve the tremendous burden borne by caretakers of the elderly long-term care population. . . . Despite unwarranted and destructive, if well-motivated, claims to the contrary, it is not as a substitute for nursing home care that community care has functioned over the past decade since its take-off in this country. It has functioned primarily, and all but exclusively, as a support system for family caretakers. It is a palliative for patients not sick enough to actually enter nursing homes (even though many nominally qualify), but sick in too many ways to be helped effectively by the episodic and medically oriented health care system we have developed in this nation.

IMPORTANCE OF NONMEDICAL CAREGIVERS

There is an enormous, rapidly growing literature on caregivers; yet it is striking how little of this literature is about the relationship between physicians and caregivers. In many ways this is justified. Most of the care at home is nonmedical and should not be "medicalized." The dominant issues are social: family relationships and neighborhood networks, caregiver stress, financing, housing, respite care, day care, transportation, and access to institutional care if needed. Physicians may have been omitted because they have not consistently fulfilled their side of the implied social contract with the caregivers of their home care patients.

A small descriptive study of caregivers, nurses, and geriatric physicians provided semi-quantitative data about the relationship between home care professionals and caregivers.[2] These professionals did not treat the patients assisted by study caregivers, reducing potential bias. Detailed interviews were conducted. None of the 12 caregivers reported being prepared by physicians for the caregiving role. This is understandable: caregiving often begins with an acute illness, during which other professionals teach caregivers. During home nursing care all caregivers reported access to nurses for advice. Once nursing ended, the picture changed. Half the caregivers reported having no professional to call for advice. Only a third reported that the physician was available. Three quarters believed physicians were not interested in the caregivers' day-to-day problems. Two of four physicians concurred, placing the emphasis for this aspect of home care on home health nurses. McCann writes:

> Caregivers and health professionals held paradoxical views regarding long-term home care. Nurses and physicians talked about the negative outcomes of home care resulting from the caregiver's poor judgement or inability to provide appropriate care, whereas caregivers spoke of their uncertainty when making decisions about the patient's care and their need for professional validation of their decisions. Nurses and physicians report that they instruct caregivers on how to monitor for changes in the patient's condition and what to do if changes occur; however, caregivers feel a great deal of anxiety about identifying changes that warrant action. Caregivers fear that they may not make the correct decisions and that their decisions will not be supported by health professionals. Three caregivers described episodes of being chastised by physicians and nurses for not seeking help soon enough. In some instances, however, the information nurses or physicians give is not specific enough to be useful, such as "have him drink a lot of water" or "if she seems too uncomfortable, give her another pain pill."[2]

Although they recognized subtle changes like decreased appetite, caregivers in this study had trouble interpreting such signs but were hesitant to "bother" physicians. These caregivers reported lacking ongoing contact with someone in the health care system.

After years of experience, my position is this: physician–caregiver relationships are very important in most home care situations. I do not mean to devalue relationships between other home care professionals and caregivers. When patients are receiving home health care, these relationships are often appropriately closer than relationships between caregivers and physicians. Then too, some caregivers are so capable and independent that they need little help. And there are caregivers who are unreliable despite earnest efforts to help them. This chapter is about relationships between caregivers and physicians, the need of caregivers for physicians' support and guidance,[3] physicians' need for help from caregivers when implementing medical treatment plans, and the value that good relationships add to patient care.

There is another side to this story that all office-based physicians should heed and that is much easier to understand after making house calls. Caregiving is prevalent among the office patients of primary care physicians. In a study of primary care patients aged 40 and over, 20% had caregiving responsibility.[4] Over half were caring for parents, over half were the sole caregivers, and a third lived with the care recipients. This is relevant because caregiving has repeatedly been shown to have deleterious health effects.[5,6] In one study, caring for a demented wife elevated men's blood pressures of 9 mm of mercury, a magnitude of change that would be credible in hypertension research.[7] Primary care physicians should recognize caregiving as a risk factor for caregiver health problems.

The National Association of Family Caregivers (9621 East Bexhill Drive, Kensington, MD 20895-3104) can provide additional materials referent to physician-caregiver relationships.

WHO ARE THE NONMEDICAL CAREGIVERS?

In home care, nonmedical informal caregivers do most of the work. Citing Store et al., Rivlin and Weiner summarize the issue.[8]

> Nearly 90 percent of the disabled old people who were not in nursing homes received assistance from relatives and friends, sometimes sup-

plemented by paid services. The majority of unpaid caregivers are women relatives of the disabled, usually wives, daughters, or daughters-in-law.[9] . . . Families devote enormous time and energy to the care of the elderly relatives, often at considerable emotional and physical cost. One study estimates that more than 27 million unpaid days of informal care are provided each week. Other studies suggest the large emotional and physical strain on families caring for elderly relatives.

The data, which quantify informal caregiver work, were reported by Liu.[10] Further detail is provided by Stone and Cafferata,[9] who start with a useful literature review. Among many ideas, one that rings particularly true is that a hierarchy exists among caregivers, starting with spouses (wives), then adult daughters, other family, and finally, neighbors or friends. The authors used data from the Informal Caregivers Survey, part of the 1982 National Long-Term Care Survey. The study sample of 6,393 noninstitutionalized elders represented 5.1 million persons. Of 2 million persons needing help with one or more ADLs, 1.8 million received informal caregiving. The care recipients were relatively debilitated. (See Table 5.1.)

Caregivers tend to be female (72%), averaging 57 years of age, with a third 65 or older. Most sole caregivers are spouses (55%–60%), followed by adult daughters. Three-fourths share quarters with care recipients. Family income is poor or near-poor for 31% of families and low-to-middle income for 57%. Only 10% are in the high income bracket. One third of caregivers are themselves in fair or poor health. The median duration of caregiving is between 1 and 4 years (44%), 20% reporting 5 years or more; and 80% provide unpaid assistance 7 days per week. The effort is considerable: 1–2 hours per day (57%), 3–4 hours per day (19%), and 5 or more hours per day (16%); the average is 4 hours. Work involves personal hygiene (67%), mobility (46%), and medications (53%). Help with household chores (81%), shopping and transportation (86%), and finances (49%) is also common. Caregivers have competing demands: employment (31%) or child care (20%). Of those recently employed, 9% left work to give care. Twenty percent reported reducing work hours, altering schedules, or missing work because of caregiving.

The authors divide caregivers into subsets: sole primary caregivers, primary caregivers receiving additional informal help from others, those receiving both formal and informal help, and secondary caregivers. Not surprisingly, sole primary caregivers are older, less healthy, almost always live with care recipients, and are not employed (84%). Care recipients with severe ADL deficits typically needed more than one helper. The last point

TABLE 5.1 Elderly Care Recipients (Age > 65)

Characteristic	%	Characteristic	%
Age > 75	57	Lives	
Female	60	Alone	11
Married	51	With spouse only	39
Income		With spouse/children	36
Poor/near poor	33	ADL deficits	
Low/middle	62	1–2	32
Perceived health		3–4	23
fair or poor	79	5–6	42

is echoed by a British study that showed that over half of the elderly needing help to get out of a chair received supportive care from more than one source.[11] And caregiving is hard work, as shown by Silliman and Sternberg, who dissected caregiving demands into categories: physical; time; prognosis; patient response; and burden associated with caregiving.[12]

It is obvious from Stone's data that caregiving is still largely "woman's work." Now women are returning to the work force and asking men to help with traditional homemaking responsibilities. There is concern that the supply of caregivers may dwindle. Yet one study suggests that women who work may not decrease caregiving,[13] raising concerns about stress, ill-health, and burnout. Middle-aged women in particular are shouldering caregiving burdens.[14] In my home care practice many primary caregivers are working women who are indeed under great stress. During the day they are separated from the dependent person, which creates great anxiety when that person is ill and they need support. Sexual differences are also important because of the preponderance of older women receiving long-term home care (71% at MCV Home Care). Male caregivers can be uncomfortable with bathing older female relatives and assisting with other aspects of personal hygiene or basic ADLs. Without help from personal care aides or women in the household or neighborhood, this factor can undermine the support system.

So where do physicians fit? There are many aspects of caregiving over which physicians have little control. For example, physical demands created by patient dependency often cannot be avoided. Consider MM, an obese woman who is completely immobile after several strokes. She must be turned frequently to prevent bedsores, to wash her skin, and to clean up her bowel movements. Still, the physician and the interdisciplinary team may be able to help. A Hoyer lift (freestanding hydraulic bedside lift with a body sling) or a hospital bed may lighten the load, or the patient may qualify for a personal care aid who can provide respite for a few hours each day. Sometimes other relatives need to hear directly from the physician about the patient's needs so that they will in turn honor the request of the primary caregiver for additional help.

Each situation is unique. For example, here are patients with roughly equal degrees of functional impairment. Mrs. N cared for her husband in their upper-middle-class apartment until he died. LN was demented and bedbound. Mrs. N was well educated, extremely anxious, and unhappy. She called me every week, often more than once, to discuss a litany of stresses and the lack of societal support available to her. Little changed clinically during the many months I served as LN's physician. My main role was to be Mrs. N's pressure valve.

My interactions with the families of MY and HB are different. MY is quadriplegic from spinal stenosis. She sits in a chair during the day but only with much help. HB is quadriplegic from a series of strokes; she is mute, bedfast, and fed by tube. Both have received home care for years. The caregiving is shared by daughters, who take turns. They never complain, and the patients have received magnificent care, better than in the best nursing homes. These families only call about sickness.

WORKING WITH NONMEDICAL CAREGIVERS

Improving Patient Function

One of the most rewarding strategies in an apparently impossible situation is to change the rules of the game by making the patient better and lightening the caregiver's burden. This may be done by injecting an arthritic knee, treating an unrecognized depression, finding and reversing occult hyperthyroidism, stopping antacids (which can cause diarrhea the caregiver must clean up), arranging for a geriatric evaluation and management (GEM) unit stay, or reducing a diuretic dose to make toileting needs less demanding. These are among the many fine points of medical home care practice. Here the physician is the best resource. If the physician does not pursue these ideas, the problems may never by resolved. Such interventions can be powerful enough to prevent institutionalization.

Avoiding Excessive Demands

This is another area where physicians can be particularly helpful. A patient's well-being is determined in part by the support system. As a patient advocate, the physician must understand caregivers' needs and limit requests to tasks that are truly important. At times, lacking familiarity with caregiving, physicians have prescribed regimens that are unrealistic, unreasonably complex, or unnecessary. Patient care should not be compromised, but caregivers must be considered when planning therapy. How often does the wound really need dressing? How often does the blood sugar need to be checked? What is a practical goal for diabetic treatment: short-term stability (yes) or preventing long-term complications (no)? How often are passive range-of-motion exercises needed? And so on.

It is also necessary to establish minimum standards for caregiving quality. When deciding if the threshold has been crossed by a delinquent caregiver, it is wise to use objective criteria. Examples include pill counts (reflecting incomplete medication), presence of new bedsores, poor nutritional parameters, unexplained depression or withdrawal, poor hygiene, low drug levels for medications whose blood levels can be measured, and other poor responses to therapy that should have worked.

Addressing Symptoms and Patient Behaviors

As reported by McCann, home care patients develop new problems, make complaints that are nonspecific, and undergo other changes that alarm caregivers. The physician must interpret the observations and alleviate the ones that are treatable. This is particularly relevant with demented patients, high-tech therapies, and other situations where the medical problems are mysterious to caregivers.

The main difference between this role and other longitudinal medical practices is that caregivers, rather than patients, present the complaints. Thus, caregivers take physicians' advice without being able to evaluate it by their own direct experience. For example, if an office patient has a bladder infection and I order an antibiotic, the patient will soon know if my advice was sound. If the person with the bladder infection is a demented older relative whose symptoms are nonspecific lower abdominal pain and reduced appetite, the caregiver has only secondhand information about the treatment's efficacy, gained by watching the patient respond. This can produce anxiety.

Providing Medical Insight

The issues here are diagnosis, prognosis, and comorbidity. Home care patients tend to have multiple coexisting illnesses with complex interactions and use numerous medications. It takes practice to explain these complex situations in terms that patients and caregivers will understand. The idea that treating one complaint may make another problem worse is difficult to grasp when one's relative appears ill. Pain may be helped by one arthritis pill, but kidney and heart conditions may be worsened, or gastric ulcers may develop. Conversely, an alternative pain medication will not affect the kidneys or heart but may cause constipation and magnify the chance of falls due to increased confusion. And caregivers often ask: "How long will caregiving last?" or "When will the patient die?" These questions are notoriously difficult to answer accurately. How will the patient change as the illness progresses, and what should the caregiver expect? What is "aortic stenosis" or a "blocked valve?" Physicians are best able to answer such questions.

Obtaining Home Medical Equipment and Other Services

As we have seen, physicians can authorize services and devices that can ease caregiver work. Other professionals, such as discharge planners, social workers, home health nurses, and physical or occupational therapists, often recommend the services, requiring only paperwork from physicians. Physicians should check to be sure that needs have not been overlooked and that services are appropriate. Then they must comply with administrative requirements for authorization.

While supporting caregivers, physicians must remain alert to potential abuse of goods and services. This might involve a few overly aggressive or unscrupulous vendors who urge physicians to order seat-lift chairs, home oximetry and oxygen therapy, unnecessarily elaborate wheelchairs, or other such items that I have been pressed to prescribe inappropriately. A caregiver may call, saying, "I was told we can have this equipment; all we need is your order." Some caregivers also manipulate "the system" to obtain more supplies than are really needed. Each instance must be considered with the needs of patients and caregivers foremost, erring on the side of supporting caregivers. Home care physicians should remain responsible participants in delivering cost-effective care, but helping caregivers comes first. They are doing 80% of the work at no charge.

Validating Caregiver Work

Caregivers often need encouragement, reassurance that they are doing a good job and doing everything they can. Such support is particularly vital because chronic home care patients tend to deteriorate despite everyone's best efforts, and caregivers may blame themselves. Validation of caregivers' work by physicians carries considerable value.

Forms and Letters

There are standard forms for authorizing home medical equipment or home nursing care. There is also a miscellaneous category of letters: certifying that the patient needs a first-floor apartment, certifying that a needed ambulance ride was medically necessary so that Medicare will pay the $350 bill, or stating that the caregiver's presence in the home is essential. We often perform such services at MCV Home Care.

Discouraging Dependency

Some patients and caregivers become too dependent on home care physicians. This can frustrate physicians, who recognize the phenomenon when receiving an inordinate number of phone calls about insignificant complaints. It can also be dangerous if caregivers lose the ability to assess situations and make appropriate decisions, leading to delays in seeking needed care.

Giving Permission for Institutionalization

Sometimes caregivers simply can't manage any longer, usually despite good intentions and hard work. As they place patients in nursing homes, guilt is common, with a feeling of failure and abandonment. Caregivers may find an extra 1.75 hours per day for their own needs after institutionalizing a relative.[15] The sense of coming freedom, anticipated, can be a measure of guilt. Physicians who have shared the course of home care can often alleviate this guilt with reassurance: "Caregiving is hard work; many people never have the strength to take on this type of responsibility, never mind sustaining the effort for years."

It is usually a change in patient or caregiver health that forces institutionalization. It is rarely the caregiver's "fault." Supportive discussions promote psychological healing for caregivers and are very important. In addition, families may be divided over this issue. The primary caregiver is worn out, but others in the family may oppose institutional care, even though they have not given much help. Physicians can mediate, preferably with the help of a social worker, and help to heal the family. The few who have done most of the caregiving work usually deserve the physician's loyalty in these painful struggles.

Encouraging Institutionalization

There are situations in which caregivers become overextended yet resist institutional care, whether because of neglect, self-interest of families who want to preserve an inheritance, or obvious caregiver burnout that the caregiver is denying. In such case physicians sometimes need to press for institutionalization.

HELPING CAREGIVERS WITH SELECTED MEDICAL MANAGEMENT ISSUES

Weissert and others have shown that home care should not usually be considered a means to prevent institutional care. Based on the Longitudinal Study on Aging,[16,17] changes in functional status, particularly ability to use the legs, and changes in social supports appear to force institutionalization. However, the laundry list of factors that have been associated with institutionalization includes certain medical problems with which caregivers commonly need physician help. Occasionally, institutional care is averted.

Consider the problem of dementia. Two middle-aged sons brought their elderly mother to my office for advice about increasingly aberrant behavior. She was pleasant, talkative, ambulatory, and moderately demented. Alzheimer's disease was likely. In three sessions we discussed the diagnosis, unfamiliar to these men, and the problems they might encounter. They were skeptical, though they later saw that the initial discussions were accurate. After that, much of her management was handled by phone. Occasionally, the sons came to the office. The lady wandered and required constant observation. She did not sleep at night. One son was single, and he lived with her, providing 24-hour supervision. The other handled the finances but had his own family. The first son had unmet personal needs, including a woman friend who lived nearby. The older, larger brother did not feel that the care and supervision given their mother was adequate. They fought, and the primary caregiver had a broken leg. He then asked me to mediate.

Care of demented persons is a major source of stress and expense in long-term home care[18–20] and dementia often predisposes people to nursing home placement.[21] Dementia is also prevalent, affecting about 30% of MCV Home Care patients at enrollment. Dementia adds greatly to the work load of home care physicians and to the interdependency between caregivers and physicians. Interactions center on controlling behaviors that are socially disruptive and stressful to caregivers, estimating prognosis, and later working through often painful discussions about nursing home placement or withholding interventions like CPR, tube feedings, antibiotics, surgery, or hospitalization. Controlling disruptive behaviors is especially problematic. First, behaviors like crying out, repeating things, refusing care, nocturnal wakefulness, and wandering tend to resist medication. Second, medications commonly used to control these behaviors have troublesome side effects like falls, sedation, orthostatic hypotension, confusion, and constipation. Changing the environment often works better.

The role of physicians in long-term dementia care was studied by comparing responses from 57 physicians and 47 family members.[22] The study was prompted by anecdotal caregiver accounts ranging from glowing appreciation to anger about physician unavailability; physicians indicated frustration with handling family crises and lack of helpful community resources. In descending order of difficulty, areas often considered difficult by physicians were nursing home placement; explaining the diagnosis or prognosis to families, dealing with disruptive family problems, counseling and advising families, referral to allied health or social services, determining degree of disability, obtaining a history, and doing paperwork. Medical concerns, by contrast, were much less often problematic.

Caregivers rated physicians highly in showing respect and care for demented patients and in giving and explaining a diagnosis. Intermediate ratings followed items such as understanding family needs, prognostication, completing forms, referring to specialists, responding to medical crises, and "treating the problems." In this intermediate range, 20% to 30% of caregivers considered physicians "not helpful at all." Subpar ratings were associated with facilitating nursing home placement, finding allied professionals to help families, intervening in family or behavioral crises, and making decisions about living situations and other social supports.

Eisdorfer summarized the primary care physician's role in home care for demented patients,[23] listing 12 services, paraphrased here: provide specific information about the nature and course of the illness; provide care to optimize patient function; refer to appropriate specialists; refer family to community resources, assist family in deciding about institutional care, alert family to financial and legal issues, counsel family or refer for psychological counseling, make house calls, obtain cognitive and psychological assessments of patient strengths and weaknesses to help the family plan care, develop plans for managing stress, refer to self-help groups, provide medication as needed.

Some caregivers are most stressed by verbal behaviors and wandering caused by dementia; others are more troubled by incontinence or tube feedings.[24] Urinary or fecal incontinence and failure to eat predispose patients to institutionalization in statistical models, and medical tubes are a common ingredient.

Caregivers need medical advice when dealing with incontinence and eating problems. For incontinence, physicians might suggest a commode chair or a voiding schedule, change the diuretic schedule, try drugs to inhibit bladder reactivity, or recommend diapers. Then caregivers may ask physicians to order a urinary catheter to reduce the need for changing clothes and sheets. The risks and benefits of this seemingly simple decision must be weighed, as discussed in chapter 2. The problem of feeding tubes was also discussed in that chapter. Caregivers are often anxious when a new technology is introduced in the home, particularly if the device is attached to a relative.

OTHER ISSUES INVOLVING CAREGIVERS

Like many home care services, caregiver support by physicians can probably be highly cost-effective. Consider IT, whose case I presented in chapter 2. Here I validated a "comfort care" approach that the patient herself preferred. This resulted in less use of acute care and less need for new, expensive medications. More important, IT's caregiver had a physician to call when the situation became difficult.

The caregiver had her hands full. IT's older sister lived in the house and became anxious when IT was sick. The caregiver would feel panic upon witnessing IT's apneic spells (temporary cessation of breathing), some of which were prolonged. She feared that the older sister would decompensate if IT died at home, and the caregiver feared that she was "missing something." Her instinct was to call an ambulance, generating a bill of $1,000 from the emergency encounter and possibly leading to another fruitless hospitalization. She really needed a chance to talk, reassurance that terminal care would not last forever, and advice about handling acute situations or getting extra help at home. With my support, the family could keep IT at home, where she preferred to be, with less cost to society.

Another consideration when analyzing the cost-effectiveness of caregiver support is that many caregivers are also employees. As suggested by the National Caregiver Study, home care physicians may find allies in the business community.[9] Studying 3,658 employees of a California corporation showed that 23% were providing special assistance to an older person.[25] Thirty-one percent of the caregivers lived with the care recipients. Thirty-seven percent of caregivers, compared with 23% of other employees, missed work because of family responsibilities, averaging 0.8 days in the 2 prior months. Personal phone calls during the day, quitting, being too tired to work, and leaving early were other concerns.

WHAT CAREGIVERS GIVE PHYSICIANS

Caregivers provide vital support to home care physicians. A capable caregiver makes the physician's job much easier, just as a weak caregiver confounds medical home care. Observant, sensible caregivers can be as helpful as the best trained nurses in reporting patient status and in giving care. The relationship is appropriately described as a partnership by the Council on Scientific Affairs of the American Medical Association.[26]

And then there are testimonials of appreciation, with which I will close this chapter. MCV Home Care receives many letters from grateful families, often following patients' deaths. Similar notes arrive at my office practice, but they are less frequent, perhaps because my home care patients are the ones who tend to die. Two of these treasured letters, included with permission, speak eloquently of what an experienced home care physician, nonphysician provider, or home care team can offer caregivers. I could not wish for higher praise and hope only that including these notes does not seem self-serving.

These came, respectively, from the caregiver for IT (described above) and the daughter of JL, a bright, independent Korean woman who feared the permanence of a living will. After her husband died and before the stroke that paralyzed her and deprived her of speech, JL had discussed her life values and care preferences with me. I later helped the family, who lived in another state, with some difficult choices.

From the caregiver of IT came this letter:

> Dear Dr. Boling,
> There seem to be no words sufficient to express my gratitude for all your help during the last days of my aunt's life. Somehow you seemed to know our needs even before we did. Your manner, your compassion, your thorough professionalism, your special kind of caring served as inspiration to me and indeed kept me going. You graciously assisted, so patiently and so gently with each situation that arose. Needless to say, I will never forget the experience, and I have the comfort of knowing that all my memories will be soothed by your refreshing reminder that there are still such caring people around. My entire family joins me in a heartfelt thank you.

JL's daughter wrote the following.

> Dear Dr. Boling,
> I wanted to thank you for taking care of my parents in the excellent way you did. You were everything a physician, an ideal one, could have been. My mother thought the world of you, as did my father. You took care of them physically and mentally, and your home care team was also extremely warm and caring. My mother enjoyed your visits and also liked talking to Jean and the others. You treated them and me with dignity and consideration.
>
> Since my mother had not left a living will, your advocacy of no heroic measures for her was a godsend. You had heard her express her wishes and you respected them. I would have been at a loss as to what to do. I whole-heartedly agree that her suffering should not have been prolonged by machines. The staff made her comfortable to the end and I felt reassured that she was at peace. Words cannot express the gratitude I feel for what you have done through the years, and at the end of my mother's life. I feel privileged that my parents and I have known you. May there be many more like you.

REFERENCES

1. Weissert WG. Seven reasons why it is so difficult to make community-based long term care cost-effective. *Health Serv Res.* 1985; 20:423–433.
2. McCann JJ. Long term home care for the elderly: Perceptions of nurses, physicians and primary caregivers. *QRB.* March 1988; 67–74.
3. Figueroa V, Mintz S. A guide to improving physician/caregiver relationships. *American Academy of Home Care Physicians Newsletter.* 1994; 6(2):10–11.
4. Andolsek KM, Clapp-Channing NE, Gehlbach SH, Moore I, Profitt VS, Sigmon A, Warshaw GA. Caregivers and elderly relatives: The prevalence of caregiving in a family practice. *Arch Intern Med.* 1988; 148:2177–2180.
5. Haley WE, Levine EG, Brown SL, Berry JW, Hughes GH. Psychological, social, and health consequences of caring for a relative with senile dementia. *J Am Geriatr Soc.* 1987; 35:405–411.
6. Baumgarten M, Battista RN, Infante-Rivard C, Hanley JA, Becker R, Gauthier S. The psychological and physical health of family members caring for an elderly person with dementia. *J Clin Epidemiol.* 1992; 45(1):61–70.
7. Moritz DJ, Kasl SV, Ostfeld AM. The health impact of living with a cognitively impaired elderly spouse. *Journal of Aging and Health.* 1992; 4(2): 244–267.
8. Rivlin AM, Wiener JM. *Caring for the Disabled Elderly: Who Will Pay?* Washington, DC: 1988; The Brookings Institution; p. 5.
9. Stone R, Cafferata GL, Sangl J. Caregivers of the frail elderly: A national profile. *Gerontologist.* 1987; 27:616–626.
10. Liu K, Manton KG, Liu BM. Home care expenses for the disabled elderly. *Health Care Financing Review.* 1986; 7(2):51–58.
11. Vetter NJ, Lewis PA, Llewellyn L. Supporting elderly people dependent at home. *Br Med J.* 1992; 304:1290–1292.
12. Silliman RA, Sternberg J. Family Caregiving: Impact of patient functioning and underlying causes of dependency. *Gerontologist.* 1988; 28(3):377–382.
13. Moen P, Robinson J, Fields F. Women's work and caregiving roles: A life course approach. *J Gerontol.* 1994; 49(4):S176–S186.
14. Brody EM. "Women in the middle" and family help to older people. *Gerontologist.* 1981; 21:471–480.
15. Moss MS, Lawton MP, Kleban MH, Duhamel L. Time use of caregivers of impaired elders before and after institutionalization. *J Gerontol.* 1993; 48(3):S102–S111.
16. Steinbach U. Social networks, institutionalization, and mortality among elderly people in the United States. *J Gerontol.* 1992; 47(4):S183–S190.
17. Wolinsky FD, Callahan CM, Fitzgerald JF, Johnson RJ. Changes in functional status and the risks of subsequent nursing home placement and death. *J Gerontol.* 1993; 48(3):S93–S101.

18. Weinberger M, Gold DT, Divine GW, Cowper PA, Hodgson LG, Schreiner PJ, George LK. Expenditures in caring for patients with dementia who live at home. *Am J Public Health.* 1993; 83:338–341.

19. George LK, Gwyther LP. Caregiver well-being: A multidimensional examination of family caregivers of demented adults. *Gerontologist.* 1986; 26:253–259.

20. Austrom MG, Hendrie HC. Quality of life: The family and Alzheimer's disease. *Journal of Palliative Care.* 1992; 8(3):56–60.

21. Montgomery RJV, Kosloski K. A longitudinal analysis of nursing home placement for dependent elders cared for by spouses vs. adult children. *J Gerontol.* 1994; :49(2):S62–S74.

22. Glosser G, Wexler D, Balmelli M. Physicians' and families' perspectives on the medical management of dementia. *J Am Geriatr Soc.* 1985; 33:383–391.

23. Eisdorfer C, Cohen D. Management of the patient and family coping with dementing illness. *J Fam Pract.* 1981; 12:831–837.

24. Zarit SH, Todd PA, Zarit JM. Subjective burden of husbands and wives as caregivers: A longitudinal study. *Gerontologist.* 1986; 26:260–266.

25. Scharlach AE, Boyd SL. Caregiving and employment: Results of an employee survey. *Gerontologist.* 1989; 29:382–387.

26. Council on Scientific Affairs of the American Medical Association. Physicians and family caregivers: A model for partnership. *JAMA.* 1993; 269:1282–1282.

PART *II*

Effectiveness, Organization, and Management of Home Health Care

CHAPTER 6

Is Medical Home Health Care Cost-Effective?

I mproved outcomes and cost-effectiveness are key criteria by which medical services are now judged. This chapter reviews the potential of home care to improve care, reduce costs, or both. I rely on William Weissert and other scholars who have focused on community-based long-term care, including Bogdonoff[1] and Robert and Rosalie Kane.[2] I will summarize background studies, then focus on medically ill patients and the physician's important contribution to cost-effective, worthwhile home care.

If there is one paper to read, it may be: "Seven Reasons Why It Is So Difficult to Make Community-Based Long Term Care Cost-Effective."[3] On the basis of the evidence, Weissert concludes that long-term home care should *not* be seen primarily as an alternative to institutional care. Rather, well-targeted, efficient community-based care should be part of an appropriate societal response to population needs. He writes:

> No one who visits a well-targeted, health-oriented community care program would argue that it is populated by individuals who do not need care. As a society we do little or nothing to relieve the tremendous burden borne by caretakers of the elderly long-term care population. . . . Despite unwarranted and destructive, if well-motivated, claims to the contrary, it is not as a substitute for nursing home care that community

care has functioned over the past decade since its take-off in this country. It has functioned primarily, and all but exclusively, as a support system for family caretakers. It is a palliative for patients not sick enough to actually enter nursing homes (even though many nominally qualify), but sick in too many ways to be helped effectively by the episodic and medically oriented health care system we have developed in this nation.[3]

EXPERIMENTAL DATA BEARING ON COMMUNITY-BASED LONG-TERM CARE

Weissert et al. comprehensively reviewed community-based care research between 1960 and 1987.[4] They screened 700 papers, reviewed 150 in detail, and analyzed the 27 most rigorous studies. Key concepts of the review are summarized below. Baseline rates of nursing home use were under 25% in 70% of studies, leaving little room for improvement through home care. Yet some interventions reduced nursing home use. In South Carolina, controls had a 59% rate of nursing home use, and a 16% reduction was found. This state had limited community-based care when that study started, which favored success. In most programs, financial savings from home care disappeared, as few patients used nursing homes, their stays were short, and home care was costly.

Hospitalization was more common, involving over 50% of controls in half of the trials. Several studies showed reduced admissions and inpatient days. New York's ACCESS Medicare/Medicaid program (1982–86) reported 47 less inpatient days per capita, possibly due to shortened hospital stays for patients awaiting nursing home beds. Yet effects on hospital days varied between trials, and some found increases. Benefits were offset by home care costs. ACCESS saved only $3,081 per capita despite reducing inpatient costs by $11,714.

Overall, there has been little or no improvement in home care patients' health, functional status, or survival. This likely reflects the fact that the patients are near life's end. However, strong, consistently positive effects are found in satisfaction with care, particularly among caregivers. Areas showing improvement include participation and performance in activities, social interaction, caregiver satisfaction, reduced caregiver burden, and resolution of unmet needs. On the basis of data available in 1987, Weissert recommends the following:

1. Link community care programs with nursing home preadmission screening programs.
2. Use multivariate models to estimate risk of institutionalization for subpopulations.
3. Set expenditure limits for home care based on more realistic estimates of institutional care use.
4. Tailor expectations and care plans to subgroups based on their particular needs, defined early in the course of care.
5. Try to reduce home care treatment costs by working to avoid excess capacity and employing utilization controls.
6. Focus more attention on outliers.
7. Avoid hospital use unless clearly expecting a benefit.
8. Emphasize congregate housing as a more efficient setting in which to deliver care.
9. Work to make home care services more efficient; home care reaches a point of diminishing returns in both intensity and duration.

I note that many of these community care programs have had a social focus, directed at preventing nursing home use. Only a few have had strong medical components. These different strategies might influence patient selection, patterns of care, and impact. Weissert and others recommend that community-based care be tailored to the needs of selected patient subgroups. Recently, Weissert and Hedrick revisited home care cost-effectiveness, now focusing on avoiding hospital costs as the main fiscal rationale for using community-based care.[5]

DETERMINING COST-EFFECTIVENESS PROVES ELUSIVE

To settle the debate over the cost-effectiveness of community-based care, the National Long Term Care Demonstration Project, or "Channeling," was conducted. This major study is well described in one issue of *Health Services Research* (1988:23[1]). The demonstration involved 10 sites, running between 1982 and 1984. Entry criteria are shown in Figure 6.1. Eighty-six percent of enrollees qualified on the basis of ADL impairment, averaging 2.7 impairments. There were two models: "basic," emphasizing case management and service coordination; and "financial," offering case

Age	Must be 65 or over.
Functional disabilty	Must have two moderate ADL disabilities, or three severe IADL impairments, or two severe IADL impairments and one severe ADL disability. (Cognitive or behavioral difficulties affecting individual ability to perform ADLs could count as one of the severe IADL impairments)
Unmet needs	Must need help with at least two categories of service affected by functional disabilities or m impairments for 6 months (meals, medications, housework/shopping, medical treatments at home, personal care), or have a fragile informal support system that may no longer be able to provide needed care.
Residence	Must be living in the community or (if institutionalized) certified as likely to be dis charged within 3 months; must reside within project catchment area.

Figure 6.1 Channeling demonstration eligibility criteria.

management plus limited discretionary funds to augment home care.

The population was frail, 22% being unable to perform any of five major ADLs, 53% being incontinent, and 70% having onset or worsening of serious health problems in the prior year. Almost 50% were hospitalized in the 2 months before they enrolled, and 60% already used home care. The patients were sick; nearly 30% of the controls died. Channeling proceeded according to plan. Cost limits (60% of nursing home costs) capped "financial model" discretionary services, and actual use was well below the limit. Though there were no changes in health outcomes or functional status, unmet needs were reduced, and life satisfaction increased slightly. Caregiver satisfaction increased more, but burden remained high. Yet only 13% of survivors were in nursing homes after 12 months, and only 19% of those alive at 18 months were institutionalized.

Thus, despite enrolling frail, needy people and following the study plan, Channeling "failed." The 10% drop in already low nursing home use was not significant, and use of hospitals and medical services did not change.

Total costs rose 6% in the basic model and 18% in the financial model. Several explanations are offered; the central one is targeting. Channeling was designed to reduce nursing home use, but nursing home use was low, and medically ill people enrolled, many already connected with home care. Targeting was difficult. One later analysis found that only 41% of controls had potential for long-term cost saving by offset nursing home use.[6]

Again, recall that after an initial assessment, the case management was conducted by community-based case managers. This "brokerage" approach was largely nonmedical. Physicians and their interdisciplinary teams were not part of the core intervention, possibly limiting control over medical care costs. Also, when channeling was conducted, nursing home care was underdeveloped but home care was readily available, which might blunt the program's impact. Weissert further suggests that the amount of "gap-filling" services in the financial model was too generous. With many nursing home stays being short, extra community support for extended periods, even at low levels, can overshadow savings. He urges using multivariate models to identify subgroups and targeting interventions tailor-made for these subgroups:

> Patients in home and community care are a heterogeneous lot. Some are at risk of institutionalization, others face death in a short time, still others may have potential for physical or mental functioning rehabilitation or stabilization, while others may be candidates for improved contentment or caregiver relief or satisfaction. To measure each patient against every one of these domains suggests that each is equally likely to benefit in every one of them. Yet, in reality, very few are good candidates for any one domain.[7]

A RATIONALE FOR AGGRESSIVE MEDICAL MANAGEMENT FOR THE HOMEBOUND

Throughout medical history, the house call has epitomized active physician participation in medical care at home, driven by recognized patient needs. And though U.S. house calls declined in frequency this century, there have been many initiatives that illustrate their value. Bluestone[8] and Cherkasky[9] describe the 1947 Montefiore Hospital Home Care program, a coordinated care system with social work, nursing, housekeeping, transportation, occupational and physical therapy, and medication services, plus round-the-clock primary and specialty physician care, all delivered at home. Estimated home care day costs were $3, whereas hospital day costs were $12 to $15. The hospital director, Bluestone, wrote:

> The hospital is emerging from its shell to serve as a clinical center surrounded by concentric circles of medical activity. Since we are entering a new era of medical care and returning to the possibilities of the home in relation to the hospital under far more favorable internal and external circumstances than ever before, we ought to examine the hospital position and take full advantage of our opportunities.[8]

It is still remarkable to study this example from 40 years ago: an integrated comprehensive system of care directed to efficiently meeting patients' needs and deemphasizing hospital care, concepts now in the policy vanguard.

Then in 1965, Medicare gave the elderly direct access to short-term acute and subacute home health care built on nonphysician services. Ongoing medical management was not a central part of Medicare home care, and without an advocate medical management inadvertently became a missing link in the chain of home care services. Yet across the country physicians have since recognized this gap in medical care.

In 1975, Brickner et al. wrote "The Homebound Aged: A Medically Unreached Group,"[10] describing a voluntary physician-led team, active today, that reached out from St. Vincent's Hospital into a community on lower Manhattan island. The authors relate cases in which serious medical problems were managed successfully at home.

Steel and colleagues later wrote about the Boston University Hospital Home Medical Service,[11] which provides physician care, social work, and nurse case management while coordinating other care. They described care of inner-city elderly, including 32% that were ambulatory but isolated, and 8% that were bedridden. Annually, 25% were hospitalized. Among nonagenarians, 59% were hospitalized, and 22 of 51 hospitalized persons had multiple admissions.[12] This subset averaged only 13 annual hospital days while under medical case management. Mean costs were $2,021 per patient-year in 1982, including the home medical service, standard home health care, outpatient care, laboratory, and medicines.

Richmond's history follows this pattern of recognized need. In the Richmond Home Medical Program,[13] four doctors were hired between 1905 and 1910 by the city of Richmond for $900 per year, each delivering 3,000 house calls by horse-drawn carriage. This system disappeared by 1947. In 1949 the Medical College of Virginia and the Visiting Nurse Association started a new medical home care program. Students and residents under faculty direction delivered over 9,000 house calls to 3,000 patients. This program was also dissolved in the early 1960s due to lack of financial and institutional support. Richmond City Health Department physicians then resumed making house calls to help public health nurses who found homebound patients lacking medical care. The senior Richmond City physician was near retirement in 1984 when I started the current Medical College of Virginia home care program.

Thus, history tells us of a need for medical home care, but perceived need is not enough. We must reduce costs. I am interested in care of the medically ill homebound and in physician home care, so I will build a case for active longitudinal management of these patients.

Obviously, sick patients need medical attention, but there are also economic reasons to focus medical management on medically ill homebound patients. One is that a revolving subset of these patients are high-cost outliers.[14] At $1,000 per inpatient day and $1,000 per emergency room visit (including transportation), a care delivery system could afford considerable medical care management if acute care use were thereby optimized. These high-cost outliers have been much studied. Age, illness, and functional limitations are important predictors and help us choose target populations for home care. Twelve percent of Medicare beneficiaries with three or more discharges incurred 58% of Medicare inpatient costs. Diagnoses like cancer and heart failure have strong associations with multiple admissions. Self-reported poor health, medical comorbidity, and complicated illness also predict hospital use in formal studies.

The concept of high-cost outliers spans the age spectrum. In the 1980 National Medical Care and Utilization Study, 10% of younger persons accounted for 73% of expenses for the young, and 15% of seniors incurred 79% of seniors' expenditures.[15] Chronic illness and functional limitation predicted high costs. The 1980 Medical Care Utilization and Expenditure Survey found one-third of medical costs and half of hospital costs being incurred by people with chronic functional impairment. Sixty-two percent of costs involved hospitals,[16] and more than half of the functionally limited were under age 65. Among youthful high-cost outliers, neurological injury is common. In Massachusetts, 205 severely disabled young adults averaged 0.8 hospital admissions, 10 inpatient days, and 1.5 emergency room visits.[17] Similar data on younger populations come from the private sector. A corporation of 80,000 found that fewer than 6% of health plan claimants were high-cost patients ($5,000–$25,000), yet they incurred 35% of all expenses.[18]

Hospitals have a clear interest here. Schroeder studied patients with 1976 hospital costs of over $4,000 at two hospitals. These patients accounted for 20% to 68% of hospital charges and only one case in six derived from a "catastrophic" illness. Half involved chronic illness lasting more than a year.[19] Zook and Moore also found that the most costly 13% of patients consumed as much hospital care as the other 87%.[20] Two thirds of the most costly cases involved multiple admissions; less than 20% involved one catastrophic event. They conclude: "Hospital economy measures should be targeted more precisely on those small groups of patients who require much longitudinal care or demonstrate a high probability of readmission." Further analysis showed that 60% of hospital costs involved recurrent admissions for one disease.

These studies suggest an opportunity. Another lies in physician behavior. Second only to terminal illness, physician behavior was the most important single predictor of costs in a Canadian study.[21] If physicians are encouraged and enabled to use home care, positive effects may follow.

SUBSTITUTING HOME CARE FOR ACUTE CARE

Kramer found more active medical needs in Medicare home care patients than in Medicare nursing home patients and suggested that home care might be more logically substituted for acute care than for institutional care.[22] Eggert and Friedman reviewed many studies, again strongly recommending interventions for patients with multiple hospital admissions.[23] This view was further endorsed by John Capitman,[24] and by Weinberger.[25] There is much evidence and opinion supporting the premise that home care may reduce acute care use, including one 1995 study showing a 50% reduction in readmissions for heart failure.[26]

Cost reduction can occur in several ways. One is direct substitution of home care for hospital care. Examples are use of home intravenous therapy and early discharge of sick patients to home health care, the well-documented "quicker and sicker" discharge phenomenon. Relatively unstable discharges jumped from 10% to 15% after DRG payment started.[27] Large datasets confirm a widespread increase in use of home health care,

particularly for "frail" patients, concurrent with prospective hospital payment (DRGs) and the pressure to reduce length of stay.[28]

Alternatively, longitudinal home care might allow more rapid diagnosis of serious problems with appropriate, shorter early hospitalizations.
This assumes that the home care team is not overly zealous in managing
serious problems at home for too long, a concern that may increase as
physicians use advanced home care more readily.

The danger of delaying acute care has been studied. Gonella analyzed
data from a large urban academic center and a community hospital.[29]
Patients were identified with 14 index diseases in similar stages, including pneumonia, urinary tract infection, and diabetes. Over 1,000 charts
were reviewed by expert physicians, categorizing admissions as "early"
(could have been managed as outpatient), "timely," and "late" (hospitalization delayed and patient had complications that might have been prevented). Late admissions lasted 18 days, compared with 7 days for timely
admissions. At one hospital, corresponding mean charges were $20,728
and $6,821. Across 176 admissions, the charge differential was $2.4 million. There is no guarantee that costly admissions would have been shorter
if they started earlier. Nor can we conclude that access to medical home
care would result in more timely admissions. Yet the data raise possibilities. Delayed care effects may be particularly relevant to those older
patients who defer seeking medical care for reasons of cost, lack of support, immobility,[30] or belief that their problems relate to "old age."[31]

Finally, acute care often entails consultation by multiple specialists.
Discontinuity of information, duplication of evaluations, performance of
unnecessary procedures, and assorted other inefficiencies could be avoided
by coordinated medical management, governed by someone familiar with
the patient, the home situation, and the care of frail populations.

Continuity can improve the process and outcome of acute care. In a
randomized trial, Wasson compared 256 male patients in a discontinuous
outpatient system with 520 men given continuous care.[32] Average age was
65. Only 1% had ADL deficits, and only 4% had limited mobility. Patients
averaged 6.5 annual outpatient visits. Hospital days were significantly
lower (5.6) in the continuity group than in the discontinuity group (9.1).
When admitted, length of stay was shorter for continuity patients (15 days
vs. 25 days). Fewer admissions were emergent (20% vs. 39%). Satisfaction was enhanced. Related findings were reported by Bigby.[33] Records
from an outpatient medical practice found that 59 of 686 admissions (9%)
were potentially preventable. Inadequate follow-up (28 cases) and adverse

drug reactions (24 cases) were important factors.

On the other hand, medical home care can increase costs. In the home you uncover new problems. Ramsdell found 1.7 new problems per case when performing a home assessment after a careful clinic-based evaluation.[34] Some problems were medical; others related to personal safety and may have been equally serious. For example, a hip fracture after a fall is both morbid and costly. Invariably, home care services are used more freely after in-home assessment, and home care costs rise. Weissert also found that despite increased home care, acute care costs increased in some trials. Experience and judgment are crucial to cost-effective practice in this population.

ATTEMPTS TO REDUCE HOSPITAL DAYS

Health service research has targeted the end of acute care episodes, the venue of discharge planners. For example, elderly patients admitted to the University of Pennsylvania with heart disease received enhanced discharge planning and 2 weeks of posthospital nursing case management in a randomized trial.[35] Early rehospitalization and short-term medical costs were reduced.

Similarly, Johns Hopkins tested the Post Hospital Support Program[36] between 1983 and 1985. The elderly patients all had caregivers, and most were African American widows with poverty-level incomes. Medical conditions were chronic, dependency levels were high, and needs for skilled care were great. A nurse and a social worker provided discharge planning and case management, with frequent home visits. Nurses carried only 20 cases, and case managers consulted with the patients' physicians. Two findings were noteworthy. First, combining index and subsequent admissions, there was a significant 10-day reduction, from 39 to 29 days, with estimated savings of $4,500 per patient after considering program costs ($3,000 per patient-year) and other costs. Second, there was significant caregiver strain that was not reduced by the intervention. The burden we place on caregivers in these very difficult situations by enabling and encouraging long-term home care must always be remembered. Scott and White Memorial Hospital also used comprehensive discharge planning by a gerontological nurse specialist for patients aged 75 and over.[37] This small randomized study found a 2-day shorter length of stay and 50% fewer immediate readmissions.

Even very low-cost interventions may reduce costs. In one randomized trial, 1,001 hospitalized patients who received ambulatory care in a teaching practice were categorized as being at low, medium, or high risk of readmission. High-risk patients averaged 2.2 emergency room visits in the prior 6 months and had poor health. Some patients then received an information package and coordinated posthospital nursing care, using both telephone contact and mailed reminders at a monthly cost of $5.20 per patient. The high-risk group had significantly lower inpatient costs ($535 vs. $800), with a nonsignificant reduction in total costs ($973 to $720).[38] Intervention group high-risk patients had more outpatient contacts and 32% fewer nonelective inpatient days.

At the other end of life, early hospital discharge of 39 very-low-birth-weight infants with follow-up at home by master's-prepared perinatal and neonatology nurses was shown to be cost-effective in a randomized controlled trial.[39] Clinical outcomes did not differ, but costs were reduced by $18,500 per case (26%), at a per-case intervention cost of about $600. Nurse specialists provided all of the home care, supported by hospital-based neonatologists.

EXPERIMENTAL DATA ON PHYSICIAN HOME CARE

One of the major questions I must face is whether physician home care work is cost-effective. Few studies have really focused on this issue. Of the studies reviewed by Weissert,[4] only a few specifically included medical care. Most relied on case managers to coordinate medical care but did not have patients' physician(s) on the intervention team. There are two such studies to consider.

THE ROCHESTER HOME CARE TEAM

Zimmer[40] led a randomized, controlled trial. Care was delivered to 82 patients by a special team: a nurse practitioner, a physician, and a social worker. Care was delivered to 76 controls by the usual sources of care. Team patients had 24-hour phone access to team members plus in-home medical assessments. Enrollees were homebound, had serious medical problems, did not have a physician who made house calls, and had an informal caregiver. Patients were stratified into a terminal group (prognosis of less than 3 months) and a nonterminal group (80%). Enrollment took 27 months. Data on each patient were collected for 6 months.

Health outcomes did not change, but caregiver satisfaction was much improved for team patients. Utilization appeared to differ between groups, but most differences were not statistically significant. Hospital costs were 38% lower for team patients, with reduced admission frequency (0.35 vs. 0.41 per patient) and lower length of stay (12.6 vs. 14.3 days). Team patients used 59% fewer nursing home days, but less than 10% entered nursing homes, with an average stay of only 60 days, so there was little effect on total costs. Out-of-home costs were reduced by 39% for the team patients. On the other side of the ledger, in-home costs increased 61%. Most of the increase came from personal care hours, followed by physician house calls and nursing visits. Total costs were 9% lower for team patients. With large variances in costs and small numbers of subjects, these differences were not statistically significant for the entire study group. However, one-third of the patients died within 6 months (half of these had cancer), and they had a different pattern of utilization. Zimmer reexamined the final 2 weeks of life for 21 team patients and 12 controls; team patients more often died at home, and there was a significant (31%) reduction in costs.[41]

This trial had merit. It was randomized and it captured key data needed to evaluate home-based care. There were also limitations. As in any small study, care was dependent on the behavior of a few providers. Fiscal incentives and the study's setting may also limit generalizability. Further, because of large variances, the power to detect cost differences was low. Despite these caveats and acknowledging the failure to show significant overall cost reductions, I remain intrigued by the trends.

Reflecting on this study from personal experience, it is often difficult to know in advance when a patient will enter the terminal stage of life, the time when the Rochester team seemed most cost-effective. I believe that in chronic care some level of longitudinal physician involvement is needed. Thus, when a situation deteriorates, the team can choose a prudent course, and caregivers will more readily accept their advice. The key may lie in making the longitudinal, chronic phase more efficient so that financial benefits gained during acute episodes or terminal care are not dissipated. There is no doubt in my mind that the model can work.

HINES VETERANS AFFAIRS HOSPITAL

Hughes, Cummings, et al. studied medical home care in the Hines Veterans Affairs Hospital home-based health care (HBHC) program.[42,43] This HBHC program had existed for 15 years, with a patient census of 50. The physician director of HBHC also ran the Hines intermediate care ward, providing continuity across settings. Between 1985 and 1987 the study enrolled 171 "terminally ill" patients and 244 "severely disabled" patients in a randomized trial with 6-month follow-up. Patients were limited in two or more ADLs or had a prognosis of death within 6 months, and all had caregivers.

Hughes compared 81 severely disabled controls with 119 severely disabled HBHC patients.[42] Controls received Medicare home health agency care and other customary care. The HBHC program included traditional home health disciplines, plus a physician and a dietitian. Twenty percent of the physician's time was dedicated to HBHC. One third of the HBHC group received house calls, and the physician participated in care planning for others. The patients had a mean age of 67 and were seriously ill: 18% died within 6 months, and half were hospitalized in the prior 6 months. HBHC patients received nonphysician services more often than did controls: physical therapy (73% vs. 32%), social work (80% vs. 5%), home aides (55% vs. 32%), and dietitian care (72% vs. 0%). Yet total home care visits, including all disciplines, were only slightly higher for HBHC patients (29 vs. 23).

As in other studies, health status did not change, and caregiver satisfaction increased. Home care costs increased 57%, and use of private hospitals decreased. HBHC patients also used more intermediate care and less acute care at the VA hospital. Total hospital costs were 24% lower, and overall costs were 8% lower, which was not statistically significant. Cost data were skewed, with large variances that reduced the study's power.

Putting the terminally ill and disabled subsets together, the results are similar. HBHC patients received more physical therapy and more social work, dietitian, and physician care at home, but total in-home visits matched the controls. Forty-four percent died during the study. Use of intermediate care VA wards increased (3.0 days vs. 1.5 days), and use of general VA wards declined (8.5 days vs. 12.2 days). There was little use of nursing homes. Hospital days, including private hospitals, were reduced (12.8 vs. 16 days), which was not significant. Home care costs increased 88% whereas hospital costs fell 29%. Total costs were 13% lower, again a nonsignificant difference.

The Hines study had its own limitations. Some relate to the VA setting. For example, 18% of controls had no health insurance and might have had limited access to "customary home care" outside the VA. Access to the intermediate care unit was unique to the VA and may have been used preferentially by HBHC patients, given the identity of the physician director. HBHC patients were more likely to have previously used private hospitals for care (31% vs. 19%), a disproportionate opportunity for savings. As with the Rochester study, there could have been unique attributes of the team members that might not be generalizable. Finally, the apparent cost savings, achieved primarily by reduced inpatient days, were not statistically significant.

Comparing the Rochester and Hines experiences, I am struck by the similar populations—functionally impaired patients with heavy use of inpatient care and high mortality—and by the similar reduction in acute care use. Both studies are afflicted by limited power and limited generalizability, and we must ultimately acknowledge their failure to prove cost-effectiveness. However, my experience convinces me that the trends toward cost-effectiveness reflect a real benefit, obscured by methodological challenges.

HOSPICE CARE

Because terminal home care may be an area for cost savings, hospice studies are relevant. The National Hospice Study included 833 patients in home-based hospices, 624 patients in hospital-based hospices, and 297 patients in conventional oncology programs deemed by peers to offer high-quality care. The main findings were these: quality of care, pain control, and patient satisfaction were comparable.[44] Hospice patients were more likely to die at home, and home-based hospice programs had a significant 32% reduction in costs compared to both conventional care and hospital-based hospices, which were roughly equivalent.

Another analysis of hospice care linked Rochester Tumor Registry data on nongeriatric cancer patients with Blue Cross claims files. Patients were grouped according to the amount of home care used in the last months of life. Those using more home care had reductions of 20% to 30% in hospital costs and total costs.[45] Caution must be exercised in drawing conclusions from administrative research that does not include direct patient assessment; still, the findings parallel other studies of home care in populations with high mortality. A common, encouraging theme of reduced costs when patients have enhanced home care during the terminal phase of life is evident. Readers should once again recall the point made by Haug in her editorial following the Rochester study, in which she cautions us not to forget caregiver burden, a hidden cost of expanding home care[46] and terminal care. I intentionally reiterate and underline this very real consideration.

LARGE-SCALE SYSTEM INTERVENTIONS

Chapter 8 describes approaches to integrated care delivery and financing that encompass ambulatory, acute, rehabilitative, home, and nursing home care. The On Lok program, now being replicated at 15 sites in the Program for All-inclusive Care of the Elderly (PACE), has succeeded in controlling costs.[47] On Lok relies on a central day health center, creative use of alternative housing, and careful supervision of all care by an interdisciplinary team, including physicians. Early data suggest that the On Lok model may be generalizable.

Another expanded system model of some interest is the Social HMO (SHMO), an extension of the Medicare HMO risk contract to include long-term care. Early results from SHMO trials have been mixed, with indications that successful linkages between acute and long-term care and systems of care for frail populations were not yet fully effective.[48] This may represent "growing pains." At the same time, conventional Medicare HMOs are expanding rapidly and developing targeted interdisciplinary team interventions for high-risk enrollees.[49] These teams are planned and often directed by geriatricians, with an active role for professional care providers. These models suggest that the marketplace and the front-line provider community have decided that this strategy makes sense when they assume financial risk.

DIFFICULTIES IN CONDUCTING MEDICAL HOME CARE RESEARCH

One reason home care research has not yet answered questions of cost-effectiveness is that the situation is very complex. One factor is population heterogeneity. Homebound patients share one common problem: immobility, with trouble accessing care. However, they also have tremendously varied needs, which affects the care process, medical outcomes, and costs. Establishing comparable control populations is particularly difficult. Studying narrowly defined subsets is one recourse. This works for specific conditions, such as management of bedsores, or single diseases like chronic lung disease.[50] However, this research approach does not address policy issues involving the entire frail population.

If the heterogeneity issue is not sufficiently challenging, it is compounded by the fact that patients change as illnesses become unstable or caregivers wear out. Homebound patients are a moving target, and they must be studied frequently. The patients' heterogeneity and the interdependency of medical outcomes with social characteristics also force one to measure many parameters. This takes much time and effort, burdens subjects, increases study costs, and complicates analyses. Here enters another measurement problem. There are validated scales for dimensions like functional status, but for many other key dimensions good tools are lacking or less suited to home care, and there is less methodological consensus among researchers.

Then there is variability of health care costs between patients, compounded by difficulty in accurately measuring costs. Home care studies try to select patients at high risk for catastrophic costs, but only a fraction incur high costs. This skews the data and mathematically reduces the power to find statistically significant differences even when real differences exist.

Home care research brings a practical complexity: researchers must travel to patients, rather than working in one place, like a hospital, nursing home, or physician office. Patients must be studied one by one, in great detail, frequently, and longitudinally. Because of cost variances, many subjects are needed to achieve statistical significance. It takes hard work and long studies to gather enough subjects. These factors combined create expensive, difficult research.

Two more issues cap this discouraging litany. First is excluding patients from the treatment group. Given an opportunity to provide care (treatment group), contrasted with a situation where access may be limited (control group), it is morally difficult to put patients in the control group. The only sound basis I have found is the rationing argument. That is, since home care programs can't enroll all of the needy within a given service area, one can justify random allocation of people to the control group. This remains emotionally difficult for those screening potential subjects.

The second issue is generalizability. Rochester and Hines were small programs, staffed by a few dedicated advocates. One was conducted in the VA system; the other was set in an area where nursing home beds were limited and the medical community was used to collaborative practice. On Lok evolved in an economically homogeneous, Medicaid-eligible, ethnically and perhaps geographically unique context. The PACE study now seeks to discover if the success of On Lok can be replicated. Excepting research that is large in scope, like Channeling and PACE, it is hard to imagine a study that would be free of concerns about generalizability. Perhaps for some combination of these reasons, home care research has lagged behind other areas of health services research in definitively answering some crucial policy questions.

SUMMING UP

Weissert is not the only scholar to caution against overly optimistic expectations of home care as a way to reduce costs. Among others, Hedrick and Inui[51] echo the inconsistency of the data, the methodological problems, and the modest benefits. Yet there is room for optimism about medical home care. Appropriate definition of subpopulations is one key. Virtually every analyst emphasizes targeting. There are types of patients who benefit more than others from medical attention during home care, and for each individual there are phases of illness during which active medical intervention is most beneficial. Research thus far has not fully explored these dimensions. Also, the world is changing, and studies are dependent on their context. To be cost-effective a medical home care system must be different from conventional care, and providers must be empowered to change the more expensive phases of care, particularly hospital and emergency care, as that becomes necessary. To close the chapter I will risk adding personal experience as a physician overseeing more than 800 home care cases to the conceptual framework I have built from formal studies.

First, I am a home care advocate. There is no doubt in my mind that home care, applied correctly by a knowledgeable team, free of perverse incentives, located in a supportive system, and aware of costs, is cost-effective. Setting aside the gratitude of patients and families, I have often seen medical, physician-led home care succeed in preventing hospitalization; in bringing patients to the hospital early enough for shorter, easier treatment of identical problems that a year before had caused long, complex admissions; in avoiding nursing home placement; and in help-ing patients recover who otherwise would have continued a life of greater functional limitation and discomfort. It pains me to read the catalog of studies that have failed to clearly demonstrate these benefits.

I am also a home care critic. I have made house calls that could have been provided by nurses but that I was forced to make because federal policy did not allow ongoing nursing care to stable patients. I have seen home care resources wasted: excess services promoted for profit; patients and caregivers manipulating the system; inept providers derailing the process of care; and home care coordinated or delivered inefficiently. Thus, I can understand those who seek to regulate and restrict home care and who have increased the bureaucracy.

Some recent initiatives have promise. One major barrier for commu-nity-based long-term care has been economic and bureaucratic compart-mentalization of resources. Acute care is loosely connected with skilled home care. Short-term home care and long-term home care run through different systems: Medicare and Medicaid. Nursing homes are often cut off from home care and acute care and may be inaccessible when there is an acute social need for alternative living arrangements, resulting in costly hospital care. Patients have financial difficulty in obtaining basic home care, and the quality is highly variable. In reporting that 35% or 40% of the work was care management, the Rochester team captures my own experience. Some of this effort is wasted on tinkering with an old, failing care delivery machine. Systems like PACE, SHMOs, and other managed care systems that contract for nursing home beds all seem to have advan-tages in organizational structure. Still, finding "proof" that these approaches work requires high-level resolve. Even now the research com-munity finds inconsistency of measurement and problems with study design that may jeopardize the validity of large future studies.

The health care environment has also changed. Hospitalizations are dra-matically shorter. Home health care is more sophisticated. Some nursing home shortages have been rectified. Adult homes, board-and-care facili-ties, senior apartment buildings, and multilevel retirement communities are all more widely used. Communities, as the context of care, are evolving.

Home care cost-effectiveness might be sensitive to the changing con-text, and medical home care may actually have greater impact now. Although inpatient stays are shorter across all ages and diagnoses, home-bound patients have illnesses that will force much inpatient care, despite good care at home. As discretionary inpatient days are weeded out, home-bound patients will be a proportionately larger part of acute care and programs that efficiently serve these patients could have proportionately more impact on acute care costs.

Another problem is the small size of medical home care teams. In a small team, efficiency is subject to short-term staffing fluctuations, provider burnout or illness, and inability to use economies of scale for administration, purchasing, or staff coverage. In a larger system that includes more individuals with home care expertise and capability, the medical home care team may function more efficiently. Nor has information technology been fully applied to medical home care. This contrasts with hospital systems that use computers for on-line management of patient records. Better data management will soon enhance home care efficiency.

Finally, experimental home care trials have been short. Weissert writes that these interventions have their greatest impact in a short period of time for any given case; there are diminishing returns. I believe that this relates in part to resource management. When the patient became permanently bedfast, did someone return the Hoyer lift to the medical equipment company, rather than continuing the rental? Did the medical team reduce its visits when the patient stabilized? Did team members avoid excessive entanglement in untractable social conflicts?

Experience tells me there is value in continuous physician involvement, but the value is often hidden. It derives from awareness of patients' situations and baseline conditions, as well as from relationships with patients and families, which later facilitate decision making when inevitable health care or social crises arrive.

Hopefully, the future will see more active exploration of the medical dimension in home care. Much of the work in long-term home care is socially driven and socially defined, and most of this work is done by unpaid caregivers. However, much of the budget for paid services involves important medical dimensions, including acute care, a substantial proportion of institutional care, and some of the home care. Weissert writes:

> We provide nursing home care with little expectation of positive outcomes and complete certainty of increased expenditures. Since most who use home and community care are frail, dependent, sick, old, alone, or a burden to caregivers, why is it not enough to provide them with care which satisfies them? We expect even less of nursing homes.[4]

Home care should be given because it is the best response to a legitimate need. Services should be targeted, customized to individuals' needs. We should require efficacy, efficiency, and limitation of resources within constraints defined at a societal level. My plea is that we reinvent and reintegrate the medical aspect of long-term home care, as a needed part of the service spectrum. From the perspective of home care research, it will take large-scale studies based on programs like PACE to foster public policy that recognizes the physician as an essential member of an interdisciplinary community care team. We can also learn from data gathered by managed care systems as they serve "difficult" populations by placing strategically defined resources in the hands of small groups of selected, well-educated providers and letting them solve the problems without first doing formal studies.

REFERENCES

1. Bogdonoff MD. Home care for frail elders: Background issues and open questions. In: Bogdonoff MD, Hughes SL, Weissert WG, Paulsen E, eds, *The Living-at-Home Program: Innovations in Service Access and Case Management.* New York, NY: Springer Publishing Company, Inc; 1991; pp. 3–8.
2. Kane RA, Kane RL. Home care and day care (pp 111–162) and Other community long-term care services (pp 163–222). In *Long-Term Care: Principles, Programs, and Policies.* New York, NY: Springer Publishing Co; 1987.
3. Weissert WG. Seven reasons why it is so difficult to make community-based long term care cost-effective. *Health Serv Res.* 1985; 20:423–433.
4. Weissert WG, Cready CM, Pawelak JE. The past and future of home and community-based long-term care. *Milbank Mem Fund Q.* 1988; 66:309–388.
5. Weissert WG, Hedrick SC. Lessons learned from research on effects of community-based long-term care. *J Am Geriatr Soc.* 1994; 42:348–353.
6. Greene VL, Lovely ME, Ondrich JI. The cost-effectiveness of community services in frail elderly population. *Gerontologist.* 1993; 33(2):177–189.
7. Weissert WG. The National Channeling Demonstration: What we knew, know now, and still need to know. *Health Serv Res.* 1988; 23:175–187.
8. Bluestone EM. The principles and practice of home care. *JAMA.* 1954; 155:1379–1382.
9. Cherkasky M. The Montefiore Hospital Home Care Program. *Am J Public Health.* 1949; 39:163–166.
10. Brickner PW, Duque T, Kaufman A, Sarg M, Jahre JA, Maturlo S, Janeski JF. The Homebound Aged: A Medically Unreached Group. *Ann Intern Med.* 1975; 82:1–6.
11. Steel K, Markson E, Crescenzi C, Hoffman S, Bissonette A. An analysis of

types and costs of health care services provided to an elderly inner-city population. *Med Care.* 1982; 20:1090–1100.

12. Patterson C, Crescenzi C, Steel K. Hospital use by the extremely elderly (nonagenarians): A two-year study. *J Am Geriatr Soc.* 1984; 32:350–352.

13. Holmes EM, Nelson K, Harper CL. The Richmond Home Medical Care Program. *Am J Public Health.* 1953; 43:596–602.

14. Ludlow R, Whitelaw N, Blum C. Description and analysis of the home-bound elderly patient under the care of a home-visit physician. *J Am Geriatr Soc.* 1992; 40(10):SA56; Abstract.

15. Garfinkel SA, Riley GF, Iannacchione VG. High-cost users of medical care. *Health Care Financing Review.* 1988; 9(4):41–52.

16. Rice DP, LaPlante MP. Medical expenditures for disability and disabling comorbidity. *Am J Public Health.* 1992; 82:739–741.

17. Meyers AR, Cupples A, Lederman RI, Branch LG, Feltin M, Master RJ, Nicastro D, Glover M, Kress D. The epidemiology of medical care utilization by severely-disabled independently-living adults. *J Clin Epidemiol.* 1988; 41:163–172.

18. Alexandre LM. High-cost patients in a fee-for-service medical plan: The case for earlier intervention. *Med Care.* 1990; 28(2):112–123.

19. Schroeder SA, Showstack JA, Roberts E. Frequency and clinical description of high-cost patients in 17 acute-care hospitals. *N Engl J Med.* 1979; 300:1306–1309.

20. Zook CJ, Moore FD. High-cost users of medical care. *N Engl J Med.* 1980; 302:996–1002.

21. Roos NP. Predicting hospital utilization by the elderly: The importance of patient, physician, and hospital characteristics. *Med Care.* 1989; 27:905–917.

22. Kramer AM, Shaugnessy PW, Pettigrew ML. Cost-effectiveness implications based on a comparison of nursing home and home health case mix. *Health Serv Res.* 1985; 20:387–405.

23. Eggert GM, Friedman B. The need for special interventions for multiple hospital admission patients. *Health Care Financing Review.* 1988; suppl:57–67.

24. Capitman JA. Case management for long-term and acute medical care. *Health Care Financing Review.* 1988; suppl:53–55.

25. Weinberger M, Oddone E. Strategies to reduce hospital admissions: A review. *Q Rev Bul.* 1989; August:257–259.

26. Rich MW, Beckham V, Wittenberg C, Leven CL, Freedland, KE, Carney RM. A multidisciplinary intervention to prevent the readmission of elderly patients with congestive heart failure. *N Engl J Med.* 1995; 333:1190–1195.

27. Kosecoff J, Kahn KL, Rogers WH, Reinisch EJ, Sherwood MJ, Rubenstein LV, Draper D, Roth CP, Chew C, Brook RH. Prospective payment system and impairment at discharge: The "quicker-and-sicker" story revisited. *JAMA.* 1990; 264:1980–1983.

28. Manton KG, Woodbury MA, Vertrees JC, Stallard E. Use of Medicare

services before and after introduction of the prospective payment system. *Health Serv Res.* 1993; 28:269–292.

29. Gonnella JS, Louis DZ, Zeleznik C, Turner BJ. The problem of late hospitalization: A quality and cost issue. *Academic Medicine.* 1990; 65:314–319.

30. Arling G. Interaction effects in a multivariate model of physician visits by older people. *Med Care.* 1985; 23:361–371.

31. Branch LG, Nemeth KT. When elders fail to visit physicians. *Med Care.* 1985; 23:1265–1275.

32. Wasson JH, Sauvigne AE, Mogielnicki P, Frey WG, Sox CH, Gaudette C, Rockwell A. Continuity of outpatient medical care in elderly men. *JAMA.* 1984; 252:2413–2417.

33. Bigby J, Dunn J, Goldman L, Adams JB, Jen P, Landefeld CS, Komaroff AL. Assessing the preventability of emergency hospital admissions: A method for evaluating the quality of medical care in a primary care facility. *Am J Med.* 1987; 83:1031–1036.

34. Ramsdell JW, Swart JA, Jackson JE, Renvall M. The yield of home visit in the assessment of geriatric patients. *J Am Geriatr Soc.* 1989; 37(1):17–24.

35. Naylor M, Brooten D, Jones R, Lavizzo-Mourey R, Meezy M, Pauly M. Comprehensive discharge planning for the hospitalized elderly. *Ann Intern Med.* 1994; 120:999–1006.

36. Oktay JS, Volland PJ. Post-hospital support program for the frail elderly and their caregivers: A quasi-experimental evaluation. *Am J Public Health.* 1990; 80:39–46.

37. Kennedy L, Neidlinger S, Scroggins K. Effective comprehensive discharge planning for hospitalized elderly. *Gerontologist.* 1987; 27:577–580.

38. Weinberger M, Smith DM, Katz BP, Moore PS. The cost effectiveness of intensive postdischarge care. A randomized trial. *Med Care.* 1988; 26:1092–1101.

39. Brooten D, Kumar S, Brown LP, Butts P, Finkler SA, Sachs SB, Gibbons A, Papadopoulos MD. A randomized clinical trial of early hospital discharge and home follow-up of very-low-birth-weight infants. *N Engl J Med.* 1986; 315:934–939.

40. Zimmer JG, Groth-Juncker A, McCusker J. A randomized controlled study of a home health care team. *Am J Public Health.* 1985; 75:134-141.

41. Zimmer JG, Groth-Juncker A, McCusker J. Effects of a physician-led home care team on terminal care. *J Am Geriatr Soc.* 1984; 32:288–292.

42. Hughes SL, Cummings J, Weaver F, Manheim LM, Conrad KJ, Nash K. A randomized trial of veterans administration home care for severely disabled veterans. *Med Care.* 1990; 28(2):135–145.

43. Cummings JE, Hughes SL, Weaver FM, Manheim LM, Conrad KJ, Nash K, Braun B, Adelman J. Cost-effectiveness of Veterans Administration hospital-based home care. *Arch Intern Med.* 1990; 150:1274–1280.

44. Greer DS, Mor V, Morris JN, Sherwood S, Kidder D, Birnbaum H. An alter-

native in terminal care: Results of the National Hospice Study. *J Chron Dis.* 1986; 39:9–26.

45. McCusker J, Stoddard AM. Effects of an expanding home care program for the terminally ill. *Med Care.* 1985; 25:373–385.

46. Haug MR. Home care for the ill elderly—who benefits? *Am J Public Health.* 1985; 75:127–128.

47. Kane RL, Illston LH, Miller NA. Qualitative analysis of the program of all-inclusive care for the elderly (PACE). *Gerontologist.* 1992; 32:771–780.

48. Manton KG, Newcomer R, Lowrimore GR, Vertrees JC, Harrington C. Social/health maintenance organization and fee-for-service health outcomes over time. *Health Care Financing Review.* 1193; 15(2): 173–202.

49. Kramer AM, Fox PD, Morgenstern N. Geriatric care approaches in health maintenance organizations. *J Am Geriatr Soc.* 1992; 40:1055–1067.

50. Bergner M, Hudson LD, Conrad DA, Patmont CM, McDonald GJ, Perrin EB, Gilson BS. The cost and efficacy of home care for patients with chronic lung disease. *Med Care.* 1988; 26:566–579.

51. Hedrick SC, Inui TS. The effectiveness and cost of home care: An information synthesis. *Health Serv Res.* 1986; 20:853–879.

CHAPTER 7

Home Care Management and Managed Care

F inding a single term to describe the process of planning and overseeing care of chronically ill persons has fostered much debate.
Here I will use the term *care management,* knowing that "case
management" is more commonly applied. Care management (or case management) has been the career focus of many scholars, and their work provides the underpinning of this chapter, which explores physicians' care
management work and their relationships with other care managers.

The basic process is well defined.[1] Patients with needs are identified
(case finding), the needs are evaluated (assessment), care is planned and
implemented, quality of care is monitored, needs are periodically
reassessed, and the care plan is appropriately revised. The complexities
and controversies multiply when one confronts the reality of limited
resources, and the organizational problems posed by the myriad of inter-
locking administrative systems, all of which may affect one individual's
care (Figure 7.1).

CARE MANAGEMENT: THE FINANCIAL MODEL

One can conceive of care management primarily in financial terms, with
costcontainment central. Here the manager has a fixed pool of resources

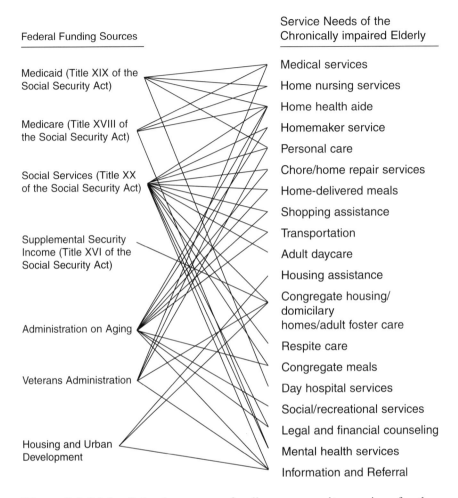

Figure 7.1 Major federal programs funding community services for the elderly.

Source: U.S. General Accounting Office: Entering a Nursing Home—Costly Implication for Medicaid and the Elderly, Washington, D.C: U.S. Government Printing Office. 1980: 74 (GAO Report No. PAD-80-12).

that are selectively allocated to meet the combined needs of many people. Service priorities follow guidelines that are necessarily political, relating individuals' needs to the population providing the shared resource. Accordingly, each payment system has idiosyncrasies. Medicare covers short-term skilled home health care but does not cover long-term basic home care. Screening mammography and hemodialysis are covered regardless of prognosis, but blood pressure medicine and dentures are not covered. A private payer may cover intravenous therapy but deny TENS (transcutaneous electrical nerve stimulation), special shoes, or knee braces.

To a large degree, political advocacy dictates allocation of resources in the financial paradigm for care management. Advocates create funding priorities. Social values also contribute to shaping allocation of shared goods. The debate over funding abortion with public monies is a case in point. Bureaucracy itself plays some role, by artificially compartmentalizing some resources and opening pipelines for others. Cost-effectiveness research has a less direct role in resource allocation decisions. This is because research data are often limited, become quickly outdated, are difficult and costly to obtain, and may not apply precisely to particular policy questions. Finally, facts are distorted by political and administrative processes that control the resources yet lack a unifying vision.

QUALITY OF CARE ISSUES UNDER THE FINANCIAL CARE MANAGEMENT PARADIGM

In a pure financial model of care management, the principal goal is cost containment, a goal that creates difficult tensions. Quality of care (see the managed care section later in this chapter) may decline as people stretch resources; provide service with substandard supplies, personnel, or oversight; or simply limit care. Virginia's Medicaid program, faced with a large state deficit in 1992, arbitrarily limited Medicaid coverage for skilled home health to 32 annual visits per patient. Payments for subsequent care of patients with serious ongoing problems were denied, straining agencies serving such patients. Special appeals were required to extend care, again increasing the burden on these agencies.

Monitoring quality is increasingly crucial as public resources are diminished and fiscal incentives tighten private sector belts. If quality erodes, an insidious process of lowering expectations follows. People rationalize as they ration, saying, "Some care is better than no care." This may be particularly familiar to home care providers in low-income urban zones or rural areas. Quality problems more often affect basic services like personal care, where pay and benefits are low and training is limited. However,

I have also seen very poor care by "skilled" providers, including physicians. Agencies that serve indigent populations may have less opportunity to train, reward, and retain experienced staff. Also, although public agencies attract some talented altruists, many highly qualified workers prefer not to work in poverty zones. Ultimately, the providers in less desirable areas tend to have fewer resources, and their patients generally have less financial help from families. Thus, the providers may be forced to choose between giving some service and giving no service.

For example, a nurse practitioner on my team called me to see a middle-aged diabetic woman, paralyzed by a stroke and confined to bed and chair for 5 years. The family had built a one-room dry-wall apartment in the dimly lit basement of their house, which is in a low-income area. The room was furnished with a hospital bed and geriatric chair. The patient had an old black-and-white TV, which she watched all day despite poor reception, a beloved stuffed dog, and liberal access to doughnuts and peanut butter. Two bright grandchildren were frequent visitors. A personal care aide from a professional agency was assigned 5 hours per day under Medicaid. Her work was monitored daily by one responsible family member and monthly by a nurse. The patient was partially aphasic but could communicate most needs. Despite her Spartan environment, she seemed happy.

The situation was stable until the key family member left to help with another sick relative, entrusting care to the aide and other less responsible adults. Soon the patient had a large bedsore on her left buttock, causing her to refuse the chair and to refuse turning. Her right leg lay under her for days, in a soiled bed, and developed acute gangrene. The aide worked with her daily as the situation evolved without seeking help. Even as we hospitalized the patient to amputate the foul-smelling leg, the aide did not grasp the seriousness of the situation.

Here the family provided long-term care at low cost and with a reasonable quality of life, judged by the patient's contentment. Then the family lapsed in its responsibility. More important, the aide also failed. Had the agency been able to provide more education, had the applicant pool been more resourceful and more willing to work in basement rooms behind furnaces, and had the agency been able to hire more selectively, this terrible situation might not have developed. The patient entered a nursing home because the responsible family member was appalled by the events and no longer desired responsibility for care oversight. The aide received extra instruction and was assigned a less complex case, but she was not fired.

The private sector is not free from quality issues related to cost containment. Indemnity insurers have case managers who are scrutinized on fiscal performance, and they could unintentionally approve too little service. Under managed care, physician "gatekeepers" likewise are given incentives to reduce costs while seeking to give good care. Fuchs, the health economist, notes that services should be rendered as long as marginal benefits exceed marginal costs.[2] He observes that we are often uncertain about where individual patients fit on the cost-benefit curve, and he recognizes potential harm to physician-patient relationships from this tension.

It is unlikely that ethical clinicians would intentionally deny essential care, but some home care might be withheld as discretionary and later prove to be more important than was first recognized. It is impossible for one clinician to weigh all the pros and cons of every treatment decision, to know the costs of service options, to balance the risk-benefit equation with costs, and still get through the day. The less informed the provider making the care management decision, the more likely it is that mistakes will be made. Home care is an area where physicians are poorly informed. It arises infrequently enough in most practices to limit on-the-job learning, and data on effectiveness are sparse. Thus, home care may be an area prone to judgment errors by providers under fiscal pressure.

Quality of care enters the financial care management model chiefly through concern about market share. A certain level of quality must be attained to compete for insurance contracts or to continue receiving public funds. At best, this has an indirect influence on decision making. Even companies who compete on quality must first compete on cost.

DECISION-MAKING CONTROL
IN THE FINANCIAL PARADIGM

In a financial care management model, decisional control lies with the payer. Resources are governed from the perspective of the larger system. Decision makers are distanced from clinical concerns, even when a now schizoid physician wears a gatekeeper hat in one room and a clinical hat in another. The functions required of financial care managers require clinical background but emphasize knowledge of all service options, costs, and cost-effectiveness, plus ability to make decisions about the likelihood that a given service would substantially improve the patient's outcome or lower costs. Issues like comfort, caregiver burden, or convenience may have a lower priority.

The quicker-and-sicker hospital discharge phenomenon associated with Medicare DRGs highlights this dilemma. Cartoons show patients ushered into the street wearing hospital gowns, intravenous poles in hand. These draw humor from the awareness that informal caregivers and patients themselves are being asked to assume more responsibility for care of acute illness. The hospital is a place for healing but only for a limited time. In part, early discharge intends to enhance quality by returning patients to peaceful, familiar, nonclinical surroundings, where there are fewer rules, more privacy, better food, and less virulent bacteria. Functionality may indeed increase, and recovery may be faster. Yet informal caregivers and doctors often work harder and suffer more anxiety as a result, and out-of-pocket costs rise. In fact, controlling hospital costs is the real driving force behind the aggressive discharge plan.

PHYSICIAN PARTICIPATION AND PARTNERSHIP IN THE FINANCIAL PARADIGM

Sometimes physician involvement is essential to cost control. For example, JB was a Medical College of Virginia Home Care patient who suffered from muscular dystrophy and morbid obesity. She weighed over 400 pounds and could not reposition herself, being totally paralyzed below the waist. She left home only with the help of four men from two rescue squads, who needed an hour to move her. JB had a Hoyer lift (a pneumatic hoist to lift patients out of bed). Years ago, when she was stronger and lighter, her aide used the lift to get JB into a wheelchair. JB was now so large that two nurses rolled her part way on her side for bathing, then rolled her back. The lift had been at the home for years before I became JB's physician. Recertification papers soon came. I knew JB could not use the mobility lift, and there was virtually no hope of her recovering enough to justify the device. I asked JB about returning it. She resisted. It symbolized the possibility that she would again use her wheelchair. We agreed that I would discover the lift's cost. If it was high, we would return the lift, but we could get it back in a day if she improved. The annual rental was over $1,000, so the lift was returned.

It would have been easier for me to authorize the continued rental. I traumatized my patient, and it took work to process this symbolic event. One could argue that the process was a therapeutic reality test. Regardless, it was painful. A physician's authority was required to make the decision and work through the issues. My silent business partners were the Medicare program and the taxpayers. Unfortunately, there is no guarantee that the money I saved will support home care for other needy patients. Rather, the savings will probably go to deficit reduction. A "closed" system in which I shared financial risk more directly would increase my motivation in such cases. Ethicists have argued that physicians are bound to advocate exclusively for their patients unless the resources saved in one case are earmarked for other patients with similar needs but greater chance of benefit. Even with this premise it would be difficult to justify JB's Hoyer lift.

CARE MANAGEMENT: THE CLINICAL PARADIGM

Care management can also be conceptualized as a clinical activity in which cost containment has at most secondary importance. Here quality of care is the primary objective, measured by satisfaction of the patient and family, providing comfort, and achieving specific clinical outcomes. Control lies with the clinician and family. Cost may affect decisions by limiting the range of affordable options, but decisions center on well-being. The knowledge and skills used in this model differ somewhat from those used in the financial model.

Familiarity with resources is vital to both, but the purpose of clinical care management is matching resources to problems. Effective clinical care managers must understand costs and payment sources to avoid raising false expectations or wasting time with impossible advice. However, there is no conflict of interest. As long as there is any chance of benefit, even a small benefit, purely clinical care managers are exclusively patient advocates.

PHYSICIANS AS HOME CARE MANAGERS

Momentarily setting aside obligations to sign orders and assume legal responsibility, physicians are often uniquely positioned with respect to home care management. Authority contributes heavily. In our society, patients and families expect physicians to have the most insight regarding clinical problems and their optimal treatment. Medical knowledge is rightly the cornerstone of this authority, whether derived from longitudinal familiarity with the case or gained through more intensive care of the serious chronic diseases that affect this population. Weighing the benefits of changing therapy against the risks is a task for which physicians should be uniquely well qualified and must address for reasons both clinical and financial.[3] Physicians may then delegate the design and oversight of home care to partners: nurses, nurse practitioners, social workers, therapists or others. Still, physicians are the courts of last resort when there are unanswered questions, when new problems arise, or when patients fare poorly.

Another reason physicians must be capable managers of home care is that other skilled home care providers are now involved only intermittently under most forms of insurance. Physicians, in theory at least, remain involved continuously. I qualify this statement because not all physicians follow homebound patients closely, whereas some home health agency workers maintain active roles over long periods, providing vital service.

The American Geriatrics Society defined the physician role in care management: "Physicians should understand the principles of care management and provide medical consultation in the care management process"[4] Emphasizing patient autonomy, the position statement also said: "Patients and/or surrogates have the right to be informed of options for care and should actively participate in the formulation of the individual care plan."

Fanale further positioned physicians as a medical consultants to teams that often have more skill in care management.[5] Although physicians' medical authority is important, this does not lessen the contribution of other professionals to planning and coordinating home care. The care management strengths and weaknesses of various disciplines and the interaction between physicians and professional caregivers fill the remainder of this chapter.

OTHER HOME CARE MANAGERS

Home care team members who are more expert than physicians in a particular clinical area may assume primary responsibility for managing part of the home care plan. Therapists, nurses, and social workers can be the "first call" for many complex problems. Patients and families rely on them as experts, and they develop independent long-term relationships. Beside expertise, physicians need help because it is hard for most physicians to visit homes often enough to manage complex home care treatment plans unassisted.

Each discipline brings unique strengths. Among their many skills, physical therapists are vital when patients with newly amputated legs are fitted for prostheses and try to regain independence. Respiratory therapists devise plans for oxygen delivery and airway management for people with respiratory failure, tracheostomies, or home ventilators. Occupational therapists make homes "user-friendly" for those with serious physical limitations. And beyond the clinical details are intricate and changeable regulations, plus a huge variety of potential resources from which to choose. As home care becomes more complex and technical, care management increasingly requires a team effort.

Discussions are ongoing regarding which professionals should be care managers, what the job includes, and how multiple managers should relate to each other. In one example, this debate pits nurses against social workers.[6] Nurses, physical therapists, occupational therapists, social workers, respiratory therapists, and speech therapists working for home health agencies or home medical equipment companies clearly do some care management. The role is longitudinal for some patients (e.g., home ventilator, lifelong nutritional support) and is intermittent for others (e.g., postacute nursing care under Medicare).

Hospital-based staff, often nurses or social workers serving as discharge planners, may provide short-term care management. Long-term care management can also be the responsibility of facility-based nurses or social workers in specialized transplant units, oncology units, dialysis units, and rehabilitation medicine units, among others. External to the medical care delivery system are other care managers. Staff from an Area Agency on Aging, social service department, or Medicaid program may have important roles in coordinating care. Private care management is a new and growing field, mostly populated by social workers or gerontological nurses who provide counseling and support and who help people with complex needs negotiate the maze of bureaucracies and providers. Private care managers usually serve the more affluent since they require out-of-pocket payment.

To better define the role, Kane studied 215 care managers,[7] mostly social workers, who described their responsibilities. The social flavor of the work is evident in Table 7.1.

TABLE 7.1 Reported Responsibilities of Case Managers

Case manager responsibility	% (*N* = 251)
Prepare client care plan	99
Seek family participation in care plan	99
Monitor client in person	98
Refer clients who are ineligible	94
Perform comprehensive client assessments	92
Complete reassessments	91
Monitor clients by phone	91
Recommend service providers	84
Purchase services or authorize purchase for client	79
Calculate cost of services in care plan	75
Make nursing home placements	73
Determine initial eligibility	67
Develop unorthodox service arrangements when needed	64
Perform screening or intake	63
Complete case management for clients in other residential settings	63
Provide direct counseling	58
Transport or accompany client to appointment	43
Complete case management for clients in nursing home	40
Screen for nursing home preadmission	28
Provide direct personal care (e.g., nursing)	9

From R.A. Kane, J.B. Penrod, & H.Q. Kivnick (1993). Ethics and case management: Preliminary results of an empirical study. In R.A. Kane & A.L. Caplan (Eds.), *Ethical conflicts in the management of home care: The case manager's dilemma.* New York: Springer Publishing Co, Inc. Copyright © 1993. Reproduced by permission.

Relationships between physicians and other care managers requires experience and a delicate balance, described in Kane and Caplan's excellent book.[8] Mollica comments:

> Case managers and physicians, when possible, should be part of a team. . . . Physicians can be too authoritarian in areas where they do not have as much expertise as the case manager, and they can also be too removed from the situation and ignore chronically ill clients who are served in community care systems. Case managers need skill and training in dealing with physicians.

I would add that physicians also need training in working with care managers, as suggested by a recent study.[9]

Finally, lest we view care management as a purely professional activity, remember the informal caregiver (or patient) who is often the ultimate care manager, with the most comprehensive job description and broadest responsibility. Some caregivers are very capable care managers. They have more intimate knowledge of the case and more time to investigate options. Appropriately, they often challenge providers.

CARE MANAGEMENT BY DOMAIN

For the sake of discussion, we can divide care management into domains, each emphasizing specific knowledge and skills. Different professions can be generically assigned preeminence as care managers in these domains, according to the nature of professional education and training typical for their discipline.

Medical Decision Making

In medical decision making, the physician is the most expert, followed by professional providers (nurse practitioners, physician assistants, clinical nurse specialists), nurses, therapists, pharmacists, social workers, and other less clinical professionals such as gerontologists. Exceptions would be physicians poorly educated about home care or therapists with special clinical expertise in one particular area, such as oncology pain management.

Home Care Treatment Planning

When developing a home care treatment plan, which typically involves many decisions outside the medical concerns so familiar to physicians and other professional providers, the hierarchy would be different. Here home care nurses, who best know the regulations and understand the actual delivery of home care, are often most expert, followed by hospital home care coordinators or discharge planners, therapists, and social workers. Medical personnel like physicians often have less expertise in this area.

Resource Finding

When finding available resources is the primary issue, the social worker is often most adept. Community-based care coordinators such as those who work for Area Agencies on Aging are also strong in this domain, and physicians are often weak.

Resource Allocation

Resource allocation is the bailiwick of third-party payer personnel. Whether these are individual case managers from a private insurance company or Medicaid screeners determining the appropriate number of personal care hours, these individuals know the limits on resources and the rules by which resources are apportioned. They are also better able than clinicians or other patient advocates to separate themselves from the patient and family and view the case objectively.

From the physician's perspective, this external care manager can help in many ways, such as taking the burden of denying services off the physician's shoulders and thereby improving the therapeutic relationship between physician and patient. Another valuable contribution is introducing new ideas about cost-effective approaches. On the other hand, external care managers, bound by the rules of their "system," may become a barrier to care the physician considers important, and conflicts may develop.

The foregoing artificial separation of domains gives some understanding of the complexity of care management and defines roles by discipline. In reality, the borders between domains blur, and individuals work to their strengths when managing care; care management is a shared process. Ideally, communication between co-managers is streamlined and open, and systems are relatively closed or simple. The more completely the longitudinal care management for an individual can be concentrated in the hands of a small, knowledgeable team, the better the continuity. Then care is arranged more efficiently and configured more appropriately to individual needs. For reasons enumerated earlier, a physician should be a central figure among these co-managers of care.

Unfortunately, except for demonstration projects that break down the barriers between publicly funded programs, such integrated approaches to care management are rarely possible when patients become frail and chronically homebound. Rather, patients now move from one manager to another as they change settings (hospital, home, nursing home) and interface with the "system" in all its Machiavellian complexity. Physicians who remain actively involved through this journey are often frustrated and confused and may feel the same lack of empowerment experienced by their patients.

THE MANAGED CARE MODEL
AND HOME HEALTH CARE

Managed care is now among the hottest and most controversial concepts in medicine. The term HMO, connoting a prototypical managed care organization, can be a disparagement, representing loss of choice and restricted care for many of my colleagues, patients, and acquaintances. Yet managed care, relying on a primary care physician who is both a gatekeeper or resource manager and a provider is now the chief paradigm for changing our health care system.

BASIC CONCEPTS IN MANAGED CARE

Managed care describes a variety of strategies for cost containment and care coordination, medical insurance governance, and provider organization. HMOs are but one type of managed care. The arrangements are so varied as to defy comprehensive classification, but common models bear mention.

A staff-model HMO employs physicians on salary, enrolls patients, and defines expectations for physician performance. These physicians work at HMO centers, whereas group-model HMOs contract with independent physician group practices, who in turn may be exclusively dedicated to care of that HMO's patients or may participate with several payers. The HMO is responsible for providing or contracting for all services, including home care. Support systems may guide physicians who are managing services like home care, and HMOs use expense profiles or chart reviews to track physician performance.

Related to group-model HMOs are independent practitioner associations (IPAs). The main distinction is the tightness of the relationship between the physician practices and the managed care organization. In

IPAs physicians are more autonomous, but in both situations patients must use providers within the system, except for extreme emergencies. In all these models, costs are controlled by prospective payment (capitation) or by physician profiling (discussed below), complemented by some type of positive or negative incentive, or by a combination of these methods.

A "looser" relationship is found in preferred provider organizations (PPOs). PPOs select physicians for their networks based on geographic location, cost profiles, and physician quality, which is hard to measure. Patients retain freedom of choice but have financial incentives to use network providers. Costs are controlled by provider profiling and case management.

Some of the tightest linkages between providers and payers are found in large managed care systems such as integrated service networks (ISNs) or accountable health plans (AHPs). Here vertical integration of services is extensive, and most if not all types of services, including home care, are delivered by providers who are exclusively part of one system. Patients are linked to the system through their employer or through purchasing cooperatives and are restricted to use of providers in the system.

With this background and considering managed care as a medical insurance phenomenon, viewing the number of enrollees helps one to appreciate the magnitude of this transformation. Using a broad definition of the term HMO, nationwide enrollment in January 1996 was 59.1 million.[10] This included 3.7 million Medicare enrollees and 4.7 million Medicaid enrollees. Pure staff-model HMOs captured only 1% of HMO enrollees. Group-model plans covered 18% IPAs held 41%, and mixed plans, with both staff or group and IPA options, enrolled 33%. Moreover, managed care is not a purely urban phenomenon. Comparing rural and urban populations, a similar percentage of the local population is enrolled in HMOs. Regional and local insurance market penetration by HMOs ranges from near zero to over 60% of the population. Growth in managed care systems has been rapid where there is high market penetration.

COST-CONTAINMENT STRATEGIES
IN MANAGED CARE

HMOs use several cost-containment strategies. In managed care, physician behavior is mainly influenced by fiscal incentives governed by profiles, along with clinical practice guidelines, information, and support systems.[11] Profiling is prevalent and is now familiar to many physicians. Physicians are compared with local or national peers, examining expenditures and practice patterns by service category. Some adjustment may be made for adverse patient mix: a disproportionate number of seriously ill and thus costly patients in one provider's panel. Payers may simply exclude extreme outlier cases from the profile or use a formula based on diagnoses to weight cases by their complexity. A physician profile is shown in Figure 7.2, with the payer and physician identity removed. This payer enrolls corporate employees, a population that includes few home care recipients, so home care does not have a separate line on the profile report, being included with "other services" and in the "aggregate" category. Profiles can become a preoccupation for physicians, particularly in the early years of experience with managed care.

Another cost-containment strategy, found in mature managed care systems, is to give physicians guidelines for cost-effective care, create management support structures that facilitate physician work, and minimize perverse financial incentives to provide less care. This approach offers a more optimistic future for home care under managed care. To augment structured care pathways for particular clinical problems like strokes, managed care systems in the Medicare marketplace are using screening programs to find high-risk patients and frail elders at the time of enrollment and then directing them into specialized interventions to control costs and improve care. These range from simple geriatric consultation to full involvement of interdisciplinary home care teams.[12]

HOME CARE DELIVERY IN MANAGED CARE

Home care is organized variously by managed care systems, and the type of arrangement can influence care. Mature systems tend to have better-developed home care departments.

If the home health component is owned and operated by the managed care organization, the patient's physician may be supported by an expert home care consultant, either a physician home care medical director or an experienced home care nurse. The consultant may advocate using home care to substitute for acute care during acute illness. However, the consultant may be less strongly motivated to recommend home care when illnesses become chronic, acuity subsides, and the benefit of home care is

Average Membership for Period:			235	

Primary Care Services

	Physician		Specialty average	
	services PMPY	cost PMPY	services PMPY	cost PMPY
Capitated Services				
Eval/mgmt	1.87	42.48	2.65	66.72
Diagnosis	.12	1.32	.30	7.32
Other	.06	4.92	.07	6.12
FFS-Services	.28	2.52	.64	8.04

Referred Services

	Physician		Specialty Average	
	services PMPY	cost PMPY	services PMPY	cost PMPY
Allergy	.00	.00	.24	4.56
Cardiology	.39	15.00	.18	19.08
Cardiovasc Surgery	.03	1.08	.01	6.00
Dermatology	.28	6.24	.19	6.24
Emergency Physician	.11	6.24	.18	8.76
Ear/nose/throat	.00	.12	.12	7.32
Gastroenterology	.03	2.52	.07	12.84
General Surgery	.11	8.64	.13	21.36
Ob/gyn	.63	93.60	.54	62.64
Hematology	.22	4.08	.25	3.84
Neurology	.16	15.00	.18	10.32
Ophthalmology	.30	69.72	.18	17.28
Orthopedics	.13	6.96	.40	30.72
All Therapys	.20	10.20	.68	19.20
Radiology	1.62	71.16	1.21	110.88
Surgery, Other	.30	32.76	.10	24.96
Urology	.07	2.52	.14	10.68
Anesthesia	.11	25.92	.10	27.24
Other Med Sub Spec.	.32	11.64	.26	9.84
Other Referred Services	.78	39.60	.73	51.12
Total	**5.79**	**423.00**	**5.89**	**464.88**

PMPY=per member per year

Figure 7.2 A primary care physician profile.

less clear. Overall, an "internal" home care provider is at financial risk and may feel some pressure to constrain home care use.

If home care is provided under contract with an organization outside the managed care system, the patient's physician may have greater direct responsibility for planning and overseeing home care. There may be no other case manager. This physician may perceive risk for excessive utilization, appearing on the physician's profile, and this may influence home care decisions. Assuming that the physician's managerial capability is judged by global expenditures, or the "bottom line," home care might be seen as a source of immediate cost overruns rather than a less certain means of offsetting greater future costs. If fiscal pressure is high, services seen as discretionary might fall by the wayside. This brings us back to quality of care.

GLOBAL QUALITY OF CARE
UNDER MANAGED CARE

Quality has become a crucial concern in managed care because of cost-containment incentives.[13] Unlike fee-for-service (FFS)medicine, if a managed care contract places providers at financial risk, physicians have fewer incentives to do more and may have incentives to do less, within limits determined by patient satisfaction and medical outcomes. These changes appear to affect physician behavior, clearly reducing inpatient care.[14]

Studies have been conducted to determine whether quality is maintained when fiscal incentives are changed in this manner. Studies of geriatric care are particularly relevant, as the elderly use more home care. Yet I am constantly reminded that home care extends far beyond geriatrics. A recent Massachusetts lawsuit involved a managed care payer who reduced the home nursing care for a child with an unusual problem, citing cost-effectiveness. Managed pediatric care is expanding rapidly, yet far more is known about geriatric managed care, which will be my focus here.

In 1982 the Tax Equity and Fiscal Responsibility Act (TEFRA, P.L. 97-248) mandated evaluation of care quality in the national Medicare HMO demonstration. The studies gave evidence that quality of care, measured by specific indicators, neither deteriorated nor improved when comparing HMO care with FFS Medicare practice. For example, the rate of functional status decline did not differ after adjusting for covariates. Prior to adjustment, HMO enrollees had less baseline functional limitation and fewer hospital admissions, were healthier, and experienced less functional decline than the FFS group.[15] Likewise, care for hypertension was no different. HMO patients were seen often, examined carefully, and had appropriate lab and radiographic studies.[16] HMO patients diagnosed with colorectal cancer also underwent similar evaluations and had similar stages of illness at diagnosis.[17] Heart failure patients received comparable care, with HMO patients receiving more immediate posthospital follow-up care.[18] And finally, preventive care, such as glaucoma screening, breast examination, mammography, and rectal and pelvic examinations, was more often performed for HMO patients, particularly in staff-model HMOs.[19]

Among its limitations, the TEFRA Medicare HMO demonstration was not randomized, it allowed voluntary enrollment and disenrollment, and it may have had inherent biases. It was also designed to look broadly at common, traceable outcomes in a large population. These cautions recognized, the findings regarding overall quality of care in the HMOs were reassuring, possibly reflecting the preventive orientation and philosophy of HMOs.

HOME CARE UTILIZATION AND OUTCOMES UNDER MANAGED CARE

The story of home care utilization under managed care may be somewhat different. Shaughnessy studied home care use, quality, and cost under HMO managed care.[20,21] This prospective study gathered data reflecting care of 1,632 patients from 38 Medicare home health agencies in three categories: 9 owned by HMOs, 14 contracting with HMOs but not exclusively affiliated; and 15 FFS agencies. Patients were studied until discharge from home care, or 12 weeks from the time of starting home care, whichever came first. Outcomes included functional, physiological, cognitive, and behavioral indicators. Also evaluated were the home environment, the amount of service used, and the costs of home health care.

There were some baseline differences between the three groups. Compared with HMO patients, FFS patients were less well: more dependent in bathing, grooming, eating, medication management, and preparing meals. HMO patients admitted to HMO-owned agencies were functionally more limited than were HMO patients admitted to contract agencies but less often entered home care after hospital discharge. That is, HMO-owned agencies more often give home care that was initiated from outpatient settings.

Home care utilization differences were substantial. In the first 60 days of care, HMO patients (both HMO categories together) averaged 12.7 total visits and 3.1 weekly visits, compared with 18.8 total and 4.4 weekly visits under FFS. Comparing the two HMO groups, HMO-owned agencies had lower service volumes than HMO contract agencies. Overall, HMOs spent $428 less per home care episode, or 33% of the FFS cost. After adjusting for case-mix differences, HMO expenses remained $401 below FFS expenses.

Importantly, outcomes also differed. Compared with HMO patients, FFS patients had greater improvement on 14 of 55 parameters. The groups were similar in the other 41 outcomes. For example, improvement in eating, among patients with trouble eating, was noted for only 34% of HMO patients, contrasted with 48% of FFS patients. Outcome differences were apparent whether patients were admitted to home care from hospital or from home, and differences were consistent across most diagnoses. Interestingly, there were no differences between groups for patients receiving home health service for wound care or infusion therapy.

These findings raise concerns that HMO patients had worse outcomes because they received less home care, though a cause-and-effect relationship is not proved. The seriousness and long-term impact of the delayed recovery by some HMO patients is also unknown. Still, given concern that managed care will cause less care or lower-quality care, the data are disturbing.

Assuming that the above findings by Shaughnessy, Retchin, Brown, and others are correct, we can speculate about differences between global quality of care and the quality of home health care under Medicare managed care. Here are some possible explanations.

1. There may be a knowledge deficit. Primary care physicians may be better informed about the aspects of care measured in the TEFRA HMO study, such as blood pressure control, mammography screening, and heart failure, which affect many office patients. By contrast, fewer patients use home care. Physicians learn little about home care during medical education and training, and many physicians remain relatively poorly informed in practice.

2. One wonders if physicians or managed care organization policymakers could be concerned about the ill-defined boundaries of costs asso-

ciated with home care. It is hard to know when home care ceases to be cost-effective. These doubts may be added to concerns about lack of utilization control and lack of opportunity for direct observation as care is given. If home care is a "black box," cost issues could dominate decision making.

Home care providers generally believe that home care is a cost-containing strategy, the assumption being that home care replaces more costly services, like hospital days, ambulance rides, and emergency room visits. The validity of this assumption was considered in the preceding chapter. In selected high-tech cases, such as some patients with complex wounds, home ventilators, or home intravenous antibiotic therapy for simple cases of osteomyelitis, home care can obviously be highly cost-effective. But even in these instances, how much home care is needed, and how much is it worth?

In technologically simpler situations, the yield from services like home occupational therapy, nursing medication review, or use of the latest, more expensive wound care materials is less clear. Physicians and HMO managers must understand the capability, indications, benefits, and burdens of home care; otherwise, direct costs may be the primary consideration. Costs are king in managed care. One *must* know and control costs to succeed.

Physicians might respond differently to these concerns, depending on how the managed care incentives are structured. Consider an IPA plan where primary care physicians receive capitation for their own services and are profiled for out-of-office expenditures, risking exclusion from the network if costs rise. They may feel personally responsible for reviewing all external expenditures involving their patients. Suppose such physicians know that a home nursing visit costs $85. This could seem substantial, compared with the "value" of a physician office visit ($35–$40) or the Medicare FFS payment for a house call ($45). A course of home health care, costing $877 using Shaughnessy's pooled HMO data, might be compared to an MRI (magnetic resonance image) scan, a low-risk, high-cost item physicians and managed care payers watch carefully. Or the course of home care might be compared with an expensive hospital day potentially saved.

This physician may also mistrust the agency's motives. Under Medicare's FFS program, an annual audit of Medicare home health agencies inhibits unbridled service delivery. If an IPA contract home health agency, needing more revenue, "runs up the bill," the agency could later risk losing the IPA contract, but this may not comfort a physician under scrutiny whose profile is affected immediately. Physicians thinking this way, primarily concerned with their own risk, might order less home care.

Contrast this pessimistic scenario with a forward-thinking managed care system that encourages appropriate use of home care through clinical guidelines and proactive case management. Theoretically, the physicians would feel more comfortable and the patients would have outcomes at least as good as those under FFS medicine. Slowly, such systems appear to be developing.

The physician's position might again be different if the home health agency were itself under capitation or were owned by the managed care organization. Then the agency would be at risk for excess service. This physician might encounter reluctance to provide services rather than overabundant enthusiasm. Both physicians and home care advocates within the managed care organization might have difficulty convincing the management leadership to allocate more resources for home care. Other management sectors within the organization might then be the ones to question home care's cost-effectiveness.

Physicians might encounter similar resistance in an indemnity insurance program or PPO with an individual case management office where a case manager, usually a nurse under pressure to control costs, held the home care pursestrings. Could you manage the care without those last two physical therapy visits or the extra nursing visit to get that last prothrombin time? These are difficult questions for physicians to answer with confidence, and they can breed frustration over constraint of physician autonomy.

3. Though they are now being developed, there are few existing guidelines to use when ordering home care. This differs from common medical questions like screening mammography. Granted, there are disputes about most guidelines: should mammograms be done yearly or every other year after age 65? What is a reasonable systolic blood pressure in the elderly: 130, 150, or 170 mm of mercury? Yet, however disputed, these are far more concrete than any available home health care guidelines.

The most specific established criteria for home health care are those used by Medicare auditors who regulate home health agencies. It takes an experienced home care nurse years to fully grasp the subtleties of this complex and often changing set of rules. Then, even if one accepts Medicare's home health guidelines as valid, this level of understanding cannot be expected of practicing physicians. Perhaps only large, mature HMOs have the personnel to provide this home care expertise internally. Still, for the present they will be using guidelines developed with sparse objective data on outcomes related to home care intensity and patterns of care.

In fairness to health services researchers, one should note that reasons for uncertainty about home care indications are many, including the wide variety of problems that are encountered in an even wider variety of settings, all of which makes definitive research costly and difficult. The knowledge deficit desperately needs to be overcome, but this will take many years. Thus, managing physicians or payers must make their best case-by-case judgments about the need for home care and must periodically reassess the continued need for service.

4. Overall, home care may simply have a lower priority for managed care payers, particularly those with small Medicare populations. In the "big picture," home care and home medical equipment still involve a small fraction of cases and 1% of costs for some commercial payers. This may not be enough to warrant internal study or cost-benefit analysis by the managed care organization, given the many other priorities.

Nor is home care likely to be a strong marketing strategy. Though large home care benefits might entice healthy people trying to imagine their future needs, attracting enrollees who are already homebound would be disadvantageous. Marketing should target healthy, health-conscious people with good social supports. In the short term, if a few homebound patients became dissatisfied because of limited home care services and left the managed care system, this might be less detrimental fiscally than attracting many frail enrollees by expanding home care benefits. This is clearly a skeptical portrayal of managed care, and it may be inaccurate; but in some markets such ideas must surely surface, at least temporarily.

5. Ultimately, the most important concern is that speedy functional recovery of older patients and other less dramatic benefits of home care are not top priority items in the hierarchy of outcomes. Shaughnessy's study did not indicate earlier death or more rapid hospital readmission under HMO home care. The differences are softer, related more closely to quality of life. This is a public policy issue for our society, as it appears that we must increasingly choose among health care benefits.

SOCIAL HMOS

An example of fully internalizing risk when caring for the frail elderly is the SHMO, in which the health care organization is responsible for all ambulatory, acute, and long-term care, including institutional care. The system must be administratively fluid, arranging services for people with functional dependency as their needs change and evolve. SHMOs create mechanisms that move patients to settings most appropriate to their needs, using physicians efficiently in this process.[22]

Still, the same basic issues, home care cost-effectiveness and societal priorities, can raise their heads as SHMO costs increase. Studies finding that home care has limited power to prevent institutionalization resurface. They are balanced by experts like Weissert, who advise that home care should be carefully targeted and viewed as complementary to institutional care, involving a different subset of patients rather than being substitutive. Likewise, one hopes that strategists will hear the voices of those with anecdotal experience like mine, those who are certain that they have succeeded in keeping people happily at home, at reasonable cost, through knowledge of home care, willingness, and persistence.

IMPORTANT CONSIDERATIONS FOR MANAGED CARE HOME HEALTH SERVICES

The Medicare HMO business, its early political history reflective of a struggle over money first and quality second,[23] remains uncertain terrain. However, it appears that managed care will gradually transform the world of geriatric care as it is transforming the private insurance world. Looking back to my question—contrasting Shaughnessy's data with the TEFRA demonstration data—it may be that HMO patients' home care outcomes were worse for reasons other than receiving less home care. Or the results may have reflected a time of transition from FFS practice to capitated practice, a time when some providers and some systems had not yet developed effective mechanisms to guide home care practice.

Some things seem clear. Unsupported, the physician manager under managed care has a difficult role: deciding which services outside the physician's office are needed and whether they are delivered cost-effectively by a given provider. The physician who is not an adept resource manager may face direct financial risk under capitation or indirect risk through profiling and later exclusion from the network. The situation is particularly difficult with home care, an area where physicians are uninformed and inexperienced.

Primary care physicians therefore need help with home care utilization decisions, relying on consultants or partners plus cost and outcome data. Practice guidelines are one useful strategy. Critical paths may also help in situations where home care can be patterned. Case managers with home care expertise and employed by the managed care systems can also be excellent resources. System administrators must support home care, and effective communication is essential throughout.

The physician's administrative cost associated with home care patients must also be recognized. A primary care physician working full-time in managed care is expected to handle about 1,800 assigned patients, assuming that the panel is not dominated by geriatric patients. This is less than the 2,000 to 2,500 active cases typical of a mature FFS practice. Reasons for the difference include the expectation that primary care offices will provide services that previously were referred to specialists, plus the requirement that primary care physicians spend more time coordinating and regulating patient care. Appropriate case-mix adjustments are needed for primary care physicians in capitated systems.[24]

Compared with ambulatory patients, home care patients create much more overhead, manifested by the need to confer by phone, fax, or letter with other home care providers or families, participate in case conferences, or complete forms. In the 1990 national survey of internists and family physicians, the average number of homebound patients per physician, using a standard definition of "homebound," was 21, ranging from 0 to 500, with a standard deviation of 42. Half of the physicians had fewer than 10 homebound patients. Average respondents reported putting in between 3 and 4 hours each week on paperwork and phone calls related to home care; this is not trivial, given a 60-hour work week. The high-user subset reported 95 annual home health agency referrals. They averaged 36 homebound patients, and case management consumed 4.7 hours per week.[25]

As managed care systems enroll more frail patients, this case management burden will be great. The work should draw appropriate recognition, both through financial support for physicians with many homebound patients and support systems that unload some of the home care burden from primary care physicians. Overhead and compensation are discussed further in chapter 12, and care delivery systems are addressed in the chapter 8.

Managed care may have unique problems in rural areas.[26] Providers are often fewer in number, so competition, capitation, and profiling are less effective cost-containment mechanisms. Thus, largely rural states may have more difficulty developing managed care systems. In particular, rural home care has its own special challenges related to distances between homes. These are not unique to managed care, but they are relevant to cost containment and profiling. And limited home care options add another rural challenge to managed care. Rural physicians report using more home care than their more urban counterparts.[25] Yet rural physicians also report insufficiently available home care services in social work; occupational, speech, and physical therapy; and home medical equipment.

Urban poverty zones may likewise prove difficult for managed care, due to difficulty in recruiting qualified providers and social complications in providing care. These difficulties may be amplified in home care because going into homes is a basic requirement, and fear of personal harm or dislike for the inner-city milieu inhibits some providers.

Mature managed care systems internalize service lines and undergo vertical integration. They must then grapple with the problem of supporting house calls and home care oversight. How will the physician's role be structured? If the service model asks primary care physicians to run a brisk, structured office practice, house calls may be difficult. Unless house calls are simply discarded, which I consider unadvisable, there are two basic choices (see chapter 8 for details).

One option is to encourage primary care physicians and associated non-physician providers to make house calls when needed by giving them support and freedom from other work. This embodies a traditional principle of primary care, which is continuity, and it addresses the logistic problem of geographic dispersion. In nonurban settings it is hard to envision a home care system that is not centered in the primary care physician's office. This strategy requires having primary care physicians who are educated about home care and who are motivated, active participants. Managed care incentives certainly favor house calls. If primary care physicians and/or payers are at risk for all costs, ambulance rides and emergency room costs are steep, compared with the cost of a house call.

The other general strategy is to use home care specialists, who have specific home care expertise. Whether operating sophisticated emergency response vehicles suited to managing acute problems or providing more basic services, home care specialists could replace primary care physicians in caring for the homebound. Continuity might lapse, particularly if house calls were used intermittently for crisis response rather than for longitudinal care, but care delivery by home care specialists might be more efficient. Even supervision of traditional home health agency care could be handled by the medical director of a home health agency if preferred by the primary care physician. Thus, one might create a group of physicians specialized in home care, reimbursed through a case mix adjusted per-case rate, salary, or other cost-containing approach. The large California Kaiser managed care system has been facing these issues. Kaiser of Northern California has been using home care specialists in the San Francisco area. Kaiser of Southern California also has many homebound senior enrollees, but they are dispersed over a much larger area, and the home care specialist approach is less viable.

Finally, information management becomes critical when patients visit physicians' offices less often and care is increasingly delivered by providers remote from the managing physician. Efficiently capturing, transmitting, and organizing pertinent information requires a dedicated system. Home care information management is further addressed in chapter 8.

Regardless of the model, an educated physician working with an interdisciplinary team plus a supportive organizational structure, is needed to effectively and efficiently address the needs of this growing population: the homebound patient enrolled in managed care. Those systems that are starting to enroll larger numbers of functionally impaired, systems like Kaiser, Humana, Henry Ford, Group Health, Health Partners, EverCare, and others, are creating geriatrics departments, interdisciplinary teams, and other innovative models for care delivery. In regions where system organization is more advanced and an atmosphere of cooperation exists between payers and providers, some beneficial aspects of managed care are emerging from the background of concerns about interference with practice and limitation of care. Though not yet fully realized, managed care has the potential to solve some of the problems encountered when integrating finances and care delivery systems across the many settings where the frail receive care.

REFERENCES

1. Kane RA, Thomas CK. What is Case Management, and Why Does It Raise Ethical Issues? Chapter 1, page 3. In *Ethical Conflicts in the Management of Home Care: The Case Manager's Dilemma.* Kane RA, Caplan AL, editors. Springer Publishing Co. New York, N.Y. 1993.
2. Fuchs VR. Paying the piper, calling the tune. Chapter 17, page 350-352. In *The Health Economy.* Harvard University Press. Cambridge, Massachusetts. 1986.

3. Angell M. Cost containment and the physician. *JAMA*. 1985; 254:1203– 1207.
4. Care management: Position of the American Geriatrics Society Public Policy Committee. *J Am Geriatr Soc*. 1991; 39:429–430.
5. Fanale JE, Keenan JM, Hepburn KW, Von Sternberg T. Care management. *J Am Geriatr Soc*. 1991; 34:431–437.
6. Mundinger MO. Community based care: Who will be the care managers? *Nursing Outlook*. 1984; 32(6):294–295.
7. Kane RA, Penrod JB, Kivnick HQ. Ethics and case management: Preliminary results of an empirical study. In: Kane RA, Caplan AL, eds, *Ethical Conflicts in the Management of Home Care: The Case Manager's Dilemma*. New York, NY: Springer Publishing Co; 1993; pp 7–25.
8. Mollica RL. Care managers and providers should be friends: Turf and control in case-managed services. In: Kane RA, Caplan AL, eds, *Ethical Conflicts in the Management of Home Care: The Case Manager's Dilemma*. New York, NY: Springer Publishing Co; 1993; p. 203.
9. Messick C, Mittlermark M, Gottlieb R, Ettinger W. Physicians and case management: The weak link in the chain? *J Am Geriatr Soc*. 1992; 40(10):SA57; Abstract.
10. InterStudy. *The competitive edge*. Industry Report 6.2; October 1996; Minneapolis, MN.
11. Iglehart JK. The American health care system: Managed care. *N Engl J Med*. 1992; 327:742–747.
12. Kramer AM, Fox PD, Morgenstern N. Geriatric care approaches in health maintenance organizations. *J Am Geriatr Soc*. 1992; 40:1055–1067.
13. Hillman AL. Health maintenance organizations, financial incentives, and physicians' judgements. *Ann Intern Med*. 1990; 112:891–893.
14. Hillman AL, Pauly MV, Kerstein JJ. How do financial incentives affect physicians' clinical decisions and the financial performance of health maintenance organizations? *N Engl J Med*. 1989; 321:86–92.
15. Retchin SM, Clement DG, Rossiter LF, Brown B, Brown R, Nelson L. How the elderly fare in HMOs: Outcomes from the Medicare competition demonstrations. *Health Serv Res*. 1992; 27:651-669.
16. Preston JA, Retchin SM. The management of geriatric hypertension in health maintenance organizations. *J Am Geriatr Soc*. 1991; 39:683–690.
17. Retchin SM, Brown B. Management of colorectal cancer in Medicare health maintenance organizations. *J Gen Intern Med*. 1990; 5(March/April):110–114.
18. Retchin SM, Brown B. Elderly patients with congestive heart failure under prepaid care. *Am J Med*. 1991; 90:236–242.
19. Retchin SM, Brown B. The quality of ambulatory care in Medicare health maintenance organizations. *Am J Public Health*. 1990; 80:411–414.
20. Shaughnessy PW, Schlenker RE, Hittle DF. A Study of Home Health Care Quality and Cost Under Capitated and Fee-for-Service Payment Systems. Volume 1: Summary Report. Center for Health Care Policy Research. 1355

South Colorado Boulevard, Suite 706. Denver, Colorado 80222.

21. Shaughnessy PW, Schlenker RE, Hittle DF. Home health care outcomes under capitated and fee-for-service payment. *Home Health Care Financing Review.* 1995; 16(1):187–222.

22. Abrahams R, Von Stermberg T, Zeps D, Dunn S, Macko P. Integrating care for the geriatric patient: Examples from the social HMO. *HMO Practice.* 1992; 6(4):12–19.

23. Iglehart JK. Seconds thoughts about HMOs for Medicare patients. *N Engl J Med.* 1987; 316:1487–1492.

24. Salem-Schatz S, Moore G, Rucker M, Pearson SD. The case for case-mix adjustment in practice profiling: When good apples look bad. *JAMA.* 1994; 272:871–874.

25. Boling PA, Keenan JM, Schwartzberg J, Retchin SM, Olson L, Schneiderman M. Reported home health agency referrals by internists and family physicians. *J Am Geriatr Soc.* 1992; 40:1241–1249.

26. Kronick R, Goodman DC, Wennberg J. The marketplace in health care reform: The demographic limitations of managed competition. *N Engl J Med.* 1993; 328:148–152.

Home Health Care Delivery System Strategies and Information Management

F ew of our health care delivery systems were designed for the functionally impaired, yet many experts would agree on some basic principles for system design.

1. Care should be organized so that patients can move easily between settings, from private dwelling to nursing home or adult home, to hospital, to outpatient treatment center, to hospice, to rehabilitation unit, and to day care or community center.
2. Each setting should address the needs of the functionally impaired; for example, hospitals might have special units with a geriatric care focus.
3. Providers in each setting should understand the needs of the functionally impaired and know the full range of care settings and care delivery options.
4. Information should be shared efficiently between settings and providers to maximize continuity and quality and minimize cost. Collaboration is vital.
5. Vested interests and perverse incentives should be removed so that all providers would strive to contain costs.

6. Quality of care should be promoted throughout the system.
7. Community-based care should usually be preferred over institutional care.
8. Transportation options for both the hale and the less agile, easily accessible community care centers, and mobile providers should be key components.
9. There should be specialized services for restoring function, like geriatric evaluation units, with use targeted to those most likely to benefit.
10. In all aspects, the system should focus on individual functionality, satisfaction of patients and families, and quality of life as guiding principles.

In this hypothetical design, patients would enroll with primary care physicians who were part of a comprehensive care system. Patient and family responsibility for costs would be determined by a partially subsidized insurance mechanism with a means test for all persons, and there would be reasonable limits on benefits, defined by community-wide consensus. Volunteerism would be encouraged for less technical help like monitoring and IADL support (shopping, money management, etc.). All paid providers would accept risk-sharing arrangements.

The services and technologies needed to realize this vision exist. The main hurdles are changing financing and provider relationships, overcoming turf issues and bureaucratic compartmentalization of resources, and containing costs. Never to be forgotten in planning systems of care for the frail and the elderly is that heterogeneity increases with age. Home care patients tend to be anomalous, each situation being unique and difficult to categorize, calling for an individualized approach. Therefore, this utopian system would include interdisciplinary teams for the homebound as part of the full complement of services I find myself regularly needing when managing the care of frail patients, listed below.

• Primary care physicians, most making some house calls and all knowing how to use home care services.
• Specialists who provide occasional in-home consultation on request.
• Nonphysician professional providers in most care settings, working with physicians as associates.
• Social work and case manager support in all phases of care for selected patients.

- Acute care hospital(s), user-friendly for elders, offering emergency care, specialized units for the frail, step-down or intermediate care, and a few hospice beds.
- Geriatric evaluation units plus inpatient/outpatient and home rehabilitation services.
- Acute and (limited) chronic psychiatric care facilities with active day hospitals.
- Outpatient centers for diagnostic testing, dialysis, infusion therapy, and surgery.
- Nursing homes, geographically dispersed and culturally diverse, with modern Alzheimer's disease units and acute care capabilities.
- Less supervised settings with many pricing options like adult homes, senior apartments, and life care communities, all linked to the medical care system.
- Advanced transportation systems for both healthy and frail patients, including low-cost nonurgent ambulance service.
- Adult and child day care or community centers, with on-site medical and rehabilitative care.
- Basic support at home: personal care, companions, home visitors.
- Electronic alert systems for selected homes.
- "Checking" or monitoring services for vulnerable or isolated persons.
- Home medical equipment providers.
- Home health agency care with active, informed medical directors and physician participation on interdisciplinary teams.
- High-tech home care, including infusion therapy, home X ray, cardiac monitoring; advanced obstetrical and perinatal home care; and respiratory care, including ventilators.
- Home hospice services.
- An emergency response system with ambulances plus emergency home care vehicles capable of complete urgent care diagnostic evaluation in the home.
- Pharmacy home delivery and consultation.
- Mobile, physician-directed interdisciplinary team(s) of "home care specialists" to provide chronic management in complex cases.
- A central resource file with lists of services, eligibility criteria, and capacity.
- A standard, shared, secure patient database to support care planning and delivery.
- Efficient electronic sharing of clinical data, whether by full-fledged

electronic medical records or electronic transmission of written, printed, or word-processed records.

IN ORGANIZED SYSTEMS HOW DOES ONE DELIVER MEDICAL CARE TO FUNCTIONALLY IMPAIRED COMMUNITY DWELLERS?

There are two general approaches that make sense. One is to concentrate care recipients in one location, like a day care center. This works best for those with some functional independence who are also medically stable. For community health centers, this requires good transportation. In life care communities, transportation is less important because distances are short.

The other approach is to mobilize providers. They need to be an inter-disciplinary team, the core of which should minimally include physicians, nonphysician providers and/or nurse specialists, social workers, and home health agency personnel. Close relationships with pharmacists, home medical equipment and personal care providers, payers, and other community resources are also needed.

This team could be a single organization with a central base, simplifying communication and coordination (Figure 8.1). However, in reality, teams will usually consist of several separate, linked organizations, thus requiring enhanced communication networks and operating systems (Figure 8.2). Physicians, based in offices or hospitals, would refer patients and direct home care but would not be home health agency staff members or home care specialists. Alternatively, home care could center on the home health agency, with physicians serving mainly as consultants (Figure 8.3), a model now being tested. In all cases, active, continuous physician participation is essential.

This recalls a central question: should home care optimally be directed by primary care physicians and traditional subspecialists, or should it be delivered and managed by home care specialists? For most patients, I believe this role should remain with their usual physicians. Such patients are those with specific, limited home care needs; those who are relatively functional and can travel to the physician's office; and those severely impaired homebound patients whose physicians are committed to home care, are knowledgeable in this area, and have the time to adequately fulfill the physician home care role.

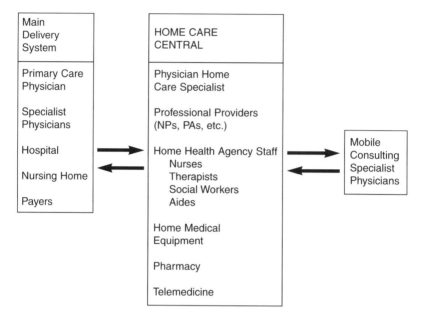

Figure 8.1 Complete home care model.

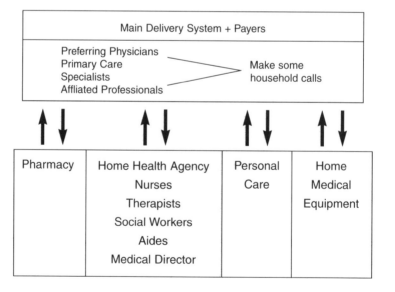

Figure 8.2 "Usual" model (physician-centered).

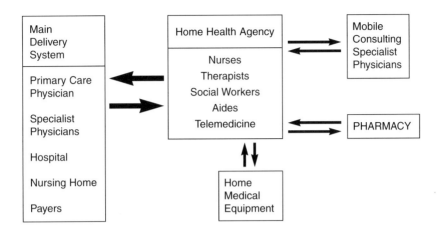

Figure 8.3 Home-health-agency-centered model.

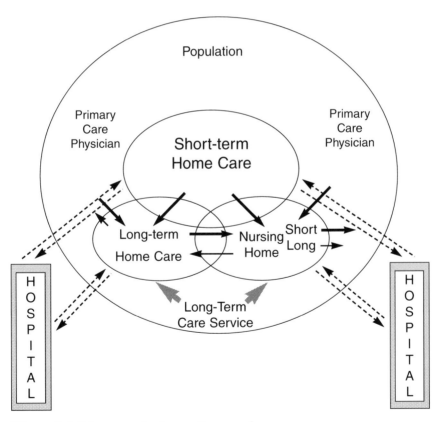

Figure 8.4 Movement in the continuum of care.

However, some home care patients need more focused attention than office-based physicians can provide. This may be due to fiscal concerns, pressure to run high-volume office practices that leave little time for home care, or lack of physician education. In Figure 8.4, these are the long-term home care patients, who, along with nursing home patients, are attended by the "long-term care service."

Here is the problem with the traditional office-based model. When patients develop complex home care problems, urgent calls from home health nurses or therapists disrupt office practices. Acute needs for physician or professional provider house calls is even more disruptive. Office-based physicians seeing patients every 15 minutes, 8 hours a day, can't have many such interruptions. One way to preserve continuity is to give office-based physicians protected time for home care work. Otherwise, complex home care must be managed by the more available medical staff of home care services who act as consultants to primary care physicians or by home care specialists who become the new primary care physicians. If one locates the home care specialists at the home health agency, strong ties to the acute medical care system must be arranged. And in any structure, good communication cannot be emphasized enough.

No matter how new systems are designed, physicians must adapt. Effective management now requires that both systems and physicians encourage patients, sometimes reluctantly, to use pathways defined by the systems. Patients have less choice of hospitals, nursing homes, specialists, or home health agencies. Physicians find themselves gently discouraging use of some "discretionary" services that patients request, recognizing them as unnecessary, or unreasonably costly. Physicians must remind patients to call before seeking emergency room care for minor ailments. The messenger carrying these messages may be exposed to anger from both patients and other providers. I have earlier discussed the role of the physician as gatekeeper, touching upon the moral, emotional, and professional quandaries this entails. The system must shelter physicians from this stress and develop positive, proactive supports, including practice guidelines, policies, and patient education.

With this conceptual framework, we can examine systems that have been built for long-term care or have added long-term care to the usual spectrum of medical services, as described in an excellent overview by Kane and Kane.[1] I will review selected model programs, focusing on the issue of continuing *medical* care.

ON LOK AND THE PACE DEMONSTRATION

Some programs incorporate several elements from my ideal long-term care program. Among the best known is San Francisco's On Lok Program for frail elders.[2] Beginning in the early 1970s, On Lok was first a day health center. Fragmentation of medical care led to addition of primary care services. On Lok now operates with combined Medicare and Medicaid funding under a Medicaid waiver and a capitation risk contract. Most enrollees are Medicaid-eligible; thus, by definition they are relatively poor.

On Lok's core is the multipurpose community center, and the model is heavily imbued with a social as opposed to a medical flavor, providing respite care and housing alternatives. Medical services provided at the center, in local hospitals, and in nursing homes are directed by On Lok physicians, who are part of an interdisciplinary team. Most in-home services involve chores and basic ADLs, rather than medical home care. On Lok has flourished, controlling medical costs and generating community support. Because of a unique relationship with the Asian community and the San Francisco setting, some questioned the potential for widespread replication of On Lok. This question is being explored in the PACE program (Progressive All-inclusive Care of the Elderly), a program for those aged 55 and over who are eligible for nursing home care.

The PACE demonstration was approved by Congress in 1986 and now involves 17 diverse sites, with a structured evaluation plan.[3] One example is the Palmetto senior care site in South Carolina. It is organized around an adult day health care center, with many on-site services. Coordinated care is provided in other settings, including the hospital, the nursing home, and the home, where physicians, nurse practitioners, social workers, pharmacists, nutritionists, and other professionals make visits as needed. The director of geriatrics, Dr. G. Paul Eleazar wrote me, saying, "Having had the opportunity to practice in multiple settings, I am firmly convinced that this model of care is *the best* for both patients and practitioners."

Such systems still lack some of the components in my utopian vision, and they depend on Medicaid funds, which restricts eligibility. PACE has grown slowly, now totaling 3,000 enrollees nationwide. PACE programs are also exclusively for the very frail, rather than being part of a system serving people with varied degrees of health and functionality. They might be considered an evolutionary form as we move toward integrated systems. We must also realize that solutions in one locality may be less successful in others, whether for reasons of geography, culture, professional territoriality, or the local economy.

THE SHMO EXPERIENCE

In 1985 the Health Care Financing Administration created a program with noncompartmentalized financing for geriatric care.[4] Pooled funds came from Medicare and Medicaid, plus patient premiums. This should permit providers to avoid some discontinuities and inefficiencies of the mainstream health care structure. Under capitation payment, SHMOs agree to deliver a full spectrum of medical and sociomedical services, including ambulatory care, acute care, and both home and institutional long-term care. The SHMO model differs importantly from the PACE model in having broader eligibility. SHMOs cannot survive if they enroll too many frail persons. They are allowed to screen applicants and limit the number of very frail enrollees, whereas PACE sites seek out frail patients eligible for nursing home care.

Abrahams, Von Sternberg, and others describe the evolution of geriatric care systems in SHMOs.[5] The hub is a case management office with a standardized assessment procedure and discretionary funds, ranging from $6,500 to $12,000 across four SHMOs, to support community-oriented long-term care. Short-term rehabilitative use of nursing homes also lies in this part of the budget. Medical instability and limited function prompt referrals to the case management office, which then integrates support services and medical services. Curiously, in the chosen example of a woman with severe heart and musculoskeletal diseases, many disciplines provided home care, but the patient still traveled monthly to the physician's office using specialized transportation.

The SHMO experience for 10,838 elderly persons enrolled in four SHMOs (Minneapolis; Portland, OR; Brooklyn; Long Beach, CA) as of June 1986 was recently compared with that of 16,664 community-dwelling seniors in the same cities.[6] The comparison was difficult because plans differ and change over time; because enrollment is voluntary, which prevents randomization and creates biases; and because the population is diverse. Moreover, 10% to 15% of enrollees switched back and forth between SHMO and several fee-for-service payers each year. To adjust for these problems, sophisticated mathematical methods were used. Data included service utilization, functional status, and other health characteristics.

The analysis suggested that SHMOs delivered basic HMO functions like ambulatory and acute care effectively, but care of impaired persons and acutely ill people with chronic illness was less effective. For very frail or demented patients, SHMOs had higher mortality rates than did fee-for-service care. Only part of the difference was explained by case mix. The authors concluded that SHMO long-term care services and their integration with acute care were still suboptimal. They commented on large case mix differences between enrolled populations and the need to adjust capitation funding rates to adequately support future SHMOs.

I would add three thoughts. First, these data reflect early experience in a transitional phase of system evolution. Later experience in mature managed care communities may be different. Second, although mortality is an important outcome, living longer does not always measure success for frail populations. Finally, the data do not include measures of enrollee or provider satisfaction, other key dimensions of quality that can be measured.

OTHER MANAGED CARE SYSTEMS

Growth in Medicare HMOs is reflected by the 1.3 million enrollees in July 1991, 2.9 million enrollees in January 1995, and 3.7 million enrollees by January 1996. In 1996 the two largest Medicare HMOs, the Secure Horizons plan in the PacifiCare system (364,818) and Kaiser Foundation Health of Northern California (265,373) enrolled 630,191 seniors.[7] At least eight states have 50,000 or more Medicare HMO enrollees[8] and by early 1996, over 10% of Medicare beneficiaries were in HMOs. Assuming that the analysts are correct and that SHMOs evolve more effectively from conventional HMOs than from long-term care systems, large Medicare HMOs are the most likely precursors to future SHMOs.

Reflecting this change, the 1996 American Geriatrics Society (AGS) meeting had a full day on managed care, the 1995 meeting was saturated with managed care presentations, and the 1994 meeting offered several abstracts and symposia on this subject. There were far fewer at the 1993 AGS meeting and virtually none in 1992. Recent abstracts in the *Journal of the American Geriatric Society* show instruments to screen populations for frailty and identify individuals at risk of high service utilization, use of interdisciplinary teams to serve high-risk individuals, extensive use of professional providers, and discussions of financing and practice organization.

Many of these strategies were noted by Kramer and Fox, who visited seven Medicare HMOs.[9] Screening for high-risk individuals relied heavily on ADLs and medication use. Management approaches included geriatric assessment units and geriatric consultation; assigning multiproblem patients to interdisciplinary teams; aggressive use of rehabilitative or subacute care in nursing homes; medication reviews; using professional providers for long-term care, mostly in nursing homes; and expanded home care, overseen by a home care coordinator.

As an example, the Kaiser plan in the San Francisco area has a group of geriatricians and home care specialists who deliver physician-directed home care. About 70 frail patients have these specialists as primary care physicians. For a larger group of several hundred patients, the home care physicians consult with and advise office-based primary care physicians during episodes of home care. By contrast, patients in the Southern California Kaiser plan are geographically dispersed. There, primary care physicians direct home care rather than using home care specialists.

Similarly, Medicaid HMOs are focusing attention on special-needs children. Although these efforts include less home care, they reflect recognition of the need to create special systems of care for selected populations.[10] This is far from being a purely geriatric issue.

LIFE CARE COMMUNITIES

Life care communities are well-suited to care of the functionally limited. A few of my patients live in such settings. The most independent live in apartments and tend to their own needs. As functional limitations develop, people move within the community to apartments designed for less independent persons, home aides are introduced, and checking services are provided. Finally, with more extreme dependency, there is nursing-home-level care.

Such communities need less medical home care. Independent patients can reach the medical office for care, with little burden on individuals and low transport costs. Social supports are more consistent, and there are fewer unknown, unpredictable factors. When in-home evaluation is needed, distances are short and patients are easy to find. Assessments by facility nurses may be accepted by patients if the nurses are familiar and trusted, reducing the need for physician house calls.

However, unless there are major changes in public long-term care policy and in the willingness of Americans to leave personal homes for retirement communities, the life care model will serve only a few of the homebound. Somers[11] projects affordability by 15% of those over age 75 in the year 2000 and by 25% in 2020. We do not yet know whether so many seniors will then choose this option. A less sophisticated, less expensive version of the life care community is the senior apartment building, which often creates socialization and social supports, with fewer "creature comforts" and with only one level of care. Medical offices may be located in these buildings, including services by professional providers.

ROCHESTER, NEW YORK: COMMUNITY-LEVEL APPROACHES

A different sort of transformation affects Rochester, New York. Set in a state known for new models of health care delivery and financing, Rochester has other key features, such as a few dominant industries, a dominant quaternary care medical center connected to community hospitals, and a dominant third-party payer, which supports community rating rather than experience rating. There is also a strong geriatrics tradition and strength in the area of medical cost-effectiveness research. Rochester's health care costs are rising more slowly than national averages, and fewer people there lack health insurance.[12] This success is attributed to planning that avoided overbedding; community-rated health insurance, a spirit of cooperation and innovation between payers and hospitals, the lack of large fee-for-service multispecialty groups; and managed care that has 65% penetration in the employed population.

Rochester is surrounded by Monroe County, home of the ACCESS program. In the early 1980s this program reported success in controlling acute care costs and making more appropriate use of nursing homes. ACCESS involved standardized assessment of individuals at high risk of nursing home placement, care planning, and limited discretionary services. Assessments traveled with patients, enhancing care coordination. Still, even in Rochester, the problem of medical care for the homebound has not been solved.

Other states, like Minnesota, have seen rapid transformation of health care financing and provider relationships, creating opportunities to improve systems.[13] Reforming health care delivery by using market forces carries some risk. Disadvantaged populations, public facilities, and medical educators are vulnerable. Also, rural areas are less suited to market-based approaches.[14] These authors favor specific local solutions.

HOME HOSPITALS

Mentioned in chapter 6 were Bluestone and Cherkasky's descriptions of the Montefiore Hospital Home Care Program, established in 1947. Montefiore offered many services at home, including generalist and specialist physician care available at all hours. The concept of a "home hospital" where serious acute illnesses are treated at home is now being rediscovered both in the United States and in Israel.[15]

A POTPOURRI

There are many other scattered accounts about home care programs. Some were funded through grants, and many have disappeared. I review a selected sampling in the following paragraphs. There are other examples; too many to mention. I find the variety of these programs refreshing and exciting, and their very existence bespeaks the compelling need. Yet their small size, impermanence, and hand-to-mouth financial existence also reflects the difficulty in providing comprehensive longitudinal home care.

The programs can be generally categorized: caregiver respite through additional short-term home care services, interventions focused on housing needs, outreach to ethnic communities with language or cultural barriers to accessing services, placing advocates in neighborhoods with many elders to help find and coordinate services, services linked to hospitals, and central databases to help people locate resources.

The urban Living-at-Home Program was beautifully described by its directors.[16] These were not medical programs, but the site development history teaches us about the complex politics of transforming health care systems. These 20 3-year community care demonstrations spanned the country, funded by the Commonwealth Fund and the Pew Charitable Trusts, with many cosponsors. Sites relied on volunteers and were only partially sustained when the grant expired. Developing each site required overcoming turf issues, as well as much planning to bring multiple agencies and providers together.

Masters' East Boston Neighborhood Health Centers program is another example. Described in chapter 3, this program helped me design the Medical College of Virginia (MCV) Home Care Program. Most care was given at neighborhood health centers (3,000 patients), with 358 patients in nursing homes and 280 patients in home care. Medical home care was provided by five nurse practitioners supported by one physician full-time equivalent (FTE). Home care nurse practitioners carried 40 to 50 cases. Along with examples from earlier chapters and those I will mention in chapter 11 ("Education for Home Health Care"), there are many reports about general or nonspecialized adult home care programs in the United States,[17,18] plus pediatric programs like those of Montefiore[19] and a Utah managed care system.[20] Reports dating back to the early 1970s include medical programs that added physician house calls to traditional home health care, as exmplified by Brickner's program at St. Vincent's Hospital in New York City.

Numerous compelling anecdotal reports and personal attestations also describe the value to both physicians and patients of physician home care work, including one by a thoracic surgeon.[21] House calls have been repeatedly endorsed,[22] along with more active physician involvement in home care,[23] by many specialty societies.[24,25] Likewise, hospitals remain interested in physician house calls. The collective weight of these accounts and expert opinions should be heeded by those planning systems of care.

Intercultural physician home care work also requires separate mention. Cultural issues in home care could fill another book, but here I would simply point to programs like the South Cove project for Oriental families in Boston, the outreach program for Spanish-speaking residents of East Harlem, and the St. Vincent's Hospital effort to help Chinese residents of lower Manhattan. In the latter example, home care physicians must learn to understand illness as being an imbalance of yin and yang, rather than using the biomedical cause-and-effect disease model that we teach in American medical education. This understanding changes the approach to therapy.[26] Providers and systems must always adapt to the cultural milieu in which people live, especially when providing home care.

INTERNATIONAL BRETHREN

The evolution of home care in the U.S. and Canadian health care systems since 1965 exhibits interesting parallels, yet compared with the United

States, Canadians spend twice as much per capita in public funds on long-term care, and they rely more heavily on institutional care. A recent student of Canada's long-term care system finds that publicly sponsored long-term care can be controlled by effective managers and administrative structures.[27] Services are directed by case managers in a single-point-of-entry system. Physician-directed medical home care programs are considered important options in Canada,[28] and physicians make four times as many chronic care visits.[29]

Likewise, medical home care programs in Britain, some targeted to older persons needing hospital care, are like those in the United States, adding support to my case when I proposed MCV Home Care to our hospital. Reports of home visiting in the Netherlands[30] and Iceland[31] add to the sense of how medical home care has been viewed in Europe, where it is a larger part of physician work.

In his book, *Adding Life to Years,* Barker describes geriatric care in Great Britain, where geriatrics and general practice figure centrally.[32] One component of integrated preventive care is the continued practice of house calls by general practitioners (GPs). For example, within the past decade virtually all Edinburgh GPs made house calls, with a median frequency of 6 to 10 per week, contrasting with the United States, where these would be annual productivity figures.[33] Yet like the United States, the British system is filled with creative local solutions to delivering community-based care rather than having a unified national strategy. In most British communities a strong nursing and social service program provides much of the care and the care coordination. GPs then offer periodic medical consultation. Barker closes by endorsing new U.S. models, like On Lok, PACE, and SHMOs, indicting the United States for lacking a health policy that supports integrated care for the elderly and warning that time is short, given the growing numbers of frail persons and rising costs.

In Israel a home care team offers comprehensive home geriatric assessment for the frail, grouping patients by need: rehabilitative, chronic maintenance, and severe debility (dementia, bedsores). The team provides longitudinal care for medically unstable chronic patients and for the extremely debilitated group while providing only short-term care for the rehabilitative group. Once patients are stable, family physicians resume care direction, using the home care team as consultants.[34] This model parallels those developing in U.S. managed care systems.

Swedish experts describe familiar debates about the marginal efficacy of home care as a substitute for institutional care.[35] Yet Swedes are developing targeted programs, like the physician-led home rehabilitation team based at the Serafen Primary Care Center in Stockholm, which shows promising evidence of cost-effectiveness.[36] The Serafen program targets patients ready for acute care hospital discharge; preventing long hospital stays is the focus.

CREATING A VIABLE SYSTEM THAT
INCLUDES MEDICAL HOME CARE

Creating new organizations that deliver efficient, comprehensive care to frail populations is fraught with difficulty. Studying the SHMO experience,[4] the PACE experience,[3] the Living-at-Home programs,[16] the nurse practitioner experience in nursing homes (see chapter 3), the community care demonstrations of the 1980s,[2] and other, similar efforts will help program developers avoid pitfalls.

Provider Workload

A key concern is provider case load. Whether one looks at PACE sites, the Rochester Home Care team; Medicare HMOs like Kaiser, Group Health, FHP, or Henry Ford Hospital; SHMOs; Living-at-Home sites; or my own MCV Home Care experience, this lesson is clear: one person, serving as the primary manager of care, can actively manage only a small number of complex home care cases. Furthermore, for each patient (or client) there should be one person—at most two closely connected people—primarily responsible for coordinating care. Caseloads depend on patient characteristics and on the context, measured in terms of both social supports for the patient and system supports for the care manager. Social factors play a huge role: at the Pasadena Living-at-Home site, 35 "difficult clients" filled one case manager's panel.

In Richmond we use a medical home care model in a population with many socioeconomic challenges, surrounded by a suboptimally integrated care system. Our nurse practitioners can handle only about 50 active cases. This is similar to the caseloads noted above and confirms information from the East Boston program, where nurse practitioners followed 40 to 50 home care patients. The MCV Home Care nurse practitioner experience also assumes ready availability of physicians and social work support. A full-time physician in our program could carry about 150 or 200 cases with help from several nurse practitioners.

Kaiser Permanente's Southern California system served 133,000 Medicare beneficiaries in a risk contract model in the summer of 1994.[37] Geriatricians' home care caseloads numbered from 52 to 130, depending on geography, admission patterns, and other responsibilities. Nurse practitioners followed from 60 to 102 patients.

British experience from the mid-1980s offers further insight into the practice capacity of primary care physicians who make house calls and direct home care.[38] These GPs had minimum requirements for a patient panel (list) of 1,000 patients and 20 clinical practice hours per week. There was an upper limit of 3,500 patients but no limit on work hours. Data derived from four separate studies. Physicians averaged 38 hours per week in general medical duties, including 24 hours of patient contact and 5 hours of travel for home visits. There were 150 office visits and 26 home visits per week. Office work consumed 18 to 20 hours, and home visits took 10 or 11 hours, including travel. Practices varied considerably. Other British observers note similar figures. In Manchester GPs saw 29 patients per day, and 12% of contacts were in patients' homes.[39] In London housecalls constituted 6% of encounters.[40]

Generally, the amount of work per complex home care patient is great, and full-time home care providers' caseloads must be small. Exceeding capacity leads quickly to poor care, provider dissatisfaction, and staff turnover. Even when such cases are a small fraction of the caseload, as is true in most office practices, one must still acknowledge the magnitude of effort required when caring for the few frail, complex patients. Otherwise, providers will avoid these cases. It is also important to realize that primary care practices age with time, so the proportion of very frail patients gradually rises. Thus, providers' roles must also change, or these patients must be moved to new systems as their needs evolve. System management must remain fluid, adaptable, and responsive to the providers.

Provider Home Care Skills

Another key issue is finding capable providers. In chapter 4 I described the skills and knowledge needed in home care as compared with nursing home work and noted some differences. A clinical example was wound care. At home the physician relies on informal caregivers, and nurses are less often present to assess wounds and change dressings, thus influencing the care plan. And it takes time for physicians to learn the administrative "ropes" and to develop referral patterns for specialized help and equipment.

Providers need exposure to different sites for community-based care. This is germane when building systems because of provider recruitment and training. House calls to private residences are not the same as adult home visits, even though the quality of care ranges from exceptional to substandard in both settings, as we know from visiting many Richmond adult homes. Adult home staffs tend to be relatively unskilled, and one must have realistic expectations about their capabilities. Experience is essential. It takes longer to gain this experience in home care than in nursing home work because it takes longer to experience the range of settings. Certain statistics bear on this point. For instance, in Missouri the distribution of patients among physicians attending nursing home patients suggests that some physicians are relatively inexperienced, whereas others follow more patients than they should.[41] Such imbalances are undesirable in a system that includes medical home care, just as one would not hire 10 cardiovascular surgeons, each doing 50 operations per year, nor one surgeon who does 500 cases.

Turf

A constant theme involving both money and pride is "turf." Almost without exception, the Living-at-Home sites described struggles by multiple social service agencies to overcome territorial issues and collaborate.[16] Similar issues confront primary care and specialist physicians, hospitals, nursing homes, and virtually every other provider in newly forming systems. Much money is involved, and historical, entrenched practice patterns of providers are rapidly changing. Providers fear losing control over their practices, their patient base, or their funding to the new organization, and they fear losing autonomy within a larger system.

Controlling the Many Phases of Care

Care managers must be able to influence care delivery throughout the system. If a chronic home care patient needs hospitalization, followed by short-term nursing home care, possibly followed by another hospital stay and more home care, a coherent plan must be developed, which then stays with the patient. MM is an example. She had acute care at two hospitals, separated by a nursing home stay, and she is now my patient at MCV Home Care again. There was little continuity. Efficient systems should not allow duplication of assessments and services, and all providers should share clinical and fiscal goals. Information handling is vital (see last section of this chapter), but collaborative relationships are the foundation that permits efficient care. Creating and maintaining such relationships requires effort.

Moving Patients Fluidly or Seamlessly

Related to information exchange is the challenge of moving patients between settings once the appropriate transition has been decided. The classic example of poor patient movement is that of a patient lying in a hospital bed for weeks or months awaiting transfer to a nursing home. New financing that combines Medicare and Medicaid funds removes barriers that have historically hindered these transitions, but other problems remain: timely availability of space in preferred settings and established referral patterns.

Changing Physicians' Roles

As care delivery systems become larger and more efficient, providers find their roles externally defined. Except in very rural areas, there is little demand for the family doctor who covers all the bases: running an office, delivering babies, setting broken bones, rounding in the hospital and the nursing home, making house calls, and doing surgery. Systems inevitably create boundaries for physicians. Some become strictly office-based, and some provide only hospital care; others staff emergency rooms. A few long-term care specialists cover nursing homes or home care. In a system, physicians relinquish some autonomy and lose some of the romantic image of the "complete physician." Continuity may diminish, which is a significant loss. Physicians, however, gain protected time and freedom from hassles, and the system benefits from predictable coverage and more efficiency. Moving from established patterns to new ways always hurts. I hear this from system developers who meet physician resistance, and I personally feel a physician's pain in both of my roles: as a traditional office-based general internist and as a new breed of home care specialist.

Finding and Keeping Staff

I will not pretend expertise in recruiting staff for ambulatory care, hospitals, or home health agencies. However, I have much experience in recruiting and retaining staff to deliver and coordinate medical home care. The available pool of qualified and motivated personnel is small, the mainstream reimbursement structure is discouraging, and the work, though rewarding, is often both physically and emotionally difficult. This makes recruitment challenging and makes team management very important. Teams are often small, so the limited pool for replacements makes turnover a very serious issue.

On Lok[2] leaders note that one key to their success has been continuity in leadership. By contrast, several PACE sites have had high turnover among day health center directors and staff physicians. Systems must create attractive and adequately funded and supported positions, to attract the staff they need for planning, delivering, and coordinating home care. System managers must listen to home care directors when they talk about burnout and caseload.

Changing Physician Attitudes

We know the common concerns of home care physicians. For example, 225 physicians listed reasons against making house calls:[42] lack of needed equipment, substandard care, cost, perceived inefficiency, and belief that many of the patients could reach the office. In the 1990 national physician home care survey,[33] 70% of physicians who did not make house calls still considered this an important service for selected patients, but 80% of them, compared with 47% of physicians who made house calls, reported being "too busy with office or hospital practice to make house calls." These attitudes call for systematic interventions, providing time and financing for home care work, plus physician education. These principles apply to both office-based home care work and house calls.

Getting Patients to Enroll

Several early studies showed trouble in getting patients to join comprehensive health care systems, leading to cash flow problems.[43] Whether because of unfamiliarity with a new concept, fear of losing choice of providers, fear of losing established relationships, or fear of "rationing," people were hesitant to join. The SHMOs each planned to enroll 4,000 elderly within 18 months. Only one succeeded in this goal by 24 months, and only two met their targets by 36 months. Delivery systems developing within existing managed care organizations performed better than systems adding managed care to long-term care organizations, perhaps reflecting experience with care management and more familiarity with managed care in certain regional populations.

Geography and Culture

When system changes envelope a region, as managed care has done on the West Coast, in Minnesota and surrounding states, and in the Northeast, shifts in cultural paradigms make it easier to create new systems. Both patients and providers become more accepting of changes wrought by the medical marketplace. Issues of culture reach deep into behavior patterns, and are regionally unique. Resources, service expectations, community practice standards, and the role of services like home care vary greatly by locale.

Similarly variable are geographic concerns and climatic conditions, as mentioned earlier. Wide-open spaces with low population density, low-income urban zones, mountains, snow, intense heat, and other factors all affect system development strategies, particularly when planning home care.

Developing Screening Criteria and Management Tools

It is important to work closely with high-risk patients from the outset. Screening instruments can identify hospital patients at risk of functional decline,[44,45] and tools can predict use of home care after hospitalization[46] or target services to prevent nursing home use.[47] Health services research provides the basis for the process. Weissert, Capitman[48] and others stress that instruments should be need-specific. The risk factor profile for recurrent medical or psychiatric hospitalization differs from that for nursing home placement or for requiring simple periodic monitoring.

Although most patients have not yet enrolled in large systems that can formally screen people and place high-risk individuals in special programs, office-based physicians can take basic steps to improve home care delivery, knowing that these will fit most developing system approaches. In the office, home care patients should be "flagged" for two reasons. One is to prompt periodic house calls. These patients are too easily overlooked or "lost to follow-up" between acute illnesses, and physicians need a "tickler" so that continuing care is given. The other reason to handle home care patients differently is administrative. Separate sections of the chart can hold copies of previous home care orders and lists of vendors or providers involved in the case. This simplifies recertification and streamlines work if new services are needed. Also useful are travel directions to the house and phone numbers of key caregivers, along with their work schedules.

Office-based physicians can reduce overhead related to home care in other ways. Earlier I wrote about preferred provider relationships and team meetings that can make home care more efficient and about proportionately reducing office staffing when physicians are on house calls. All these strategies may help office practices prepare for the approaching time when efficient physician home care will be a necessity rather than an optional, often frustrating service.

INSURANCE REFORM, SYSTEM REFORM, AND VULNERABLE POPULATIONS

Economic pressures are forcing seismic upheavals in the presently chaotic arrangement of health care financing and administration. What results will have far-reaching effects on care of the frail, most of whom cannot work and many of whom are elderly? In 1992 and 1993, Iglehart wrote an excellent series of articles for the *New England Journal of Medicine,* describing current components: Medicare, Medicaid, private insurance, and managed care. Additional out-of-pocket funding comes from private citizens. Monies from local governments support public facilities, and smaller amounts come from research grants and charitable foundations. A great uncertainty is whether the new equilibrium will be equitable or vulnerable populations will be slighted. For example, if Medicare's budget is indiscriminately slashed by 20%, as proposed in the 1995 U.S. Congress, who will ensure that my frail, sick inner-city patients can get the home care they so clearly need?

The medical marketplace defines new priorities. Although the analogy is imperfect, I recall ads by a profitable suburban hospital for a van to make house calls to new mothers. These are really nursing visits to check on the mothers during the postpartum period, which is a great idea. It is relatively inexpensive, may prevent costly problems, and is wonderful for marketing to a desirable group of potential clients: insured young women. How much friendlier could a hospital be? Staff recruitment for such jobs also should be easy.

The house calls made by my MCV Home Care staff are much different. This resource-intensive, comparatively costly program is located downtown in a public hospital. The patients are seriously ill, needing lots of continuing care. The budget is always at risk in an increasingly stringent fiscal environment. If we advertised our house calls, as the "mom's van" is promoted, we would be flooded with calls that would quickly overwhelm our meager capacity. Each new patient would increase the deficit incurred by the physicians because of low Medicare house call payment. We believe the program is cost-effective. Yet the new inpatient business we bring to the hospital does not have a large enough margin under Medicare DRGs to support widely expanding the program. Even in a large, efficient capitated system, where our cost effectiveness was accepted as an added value, we would not advertise geriatric house calls for fear of attracting costly patients to the risk pool.

Whether there is ultimately a single payer system, which I consider the likely denouement, or a collection of large competing systems, one test of our society will be the care we extend to those who are immobile. Large issues of intergenerational equity and social values arise. The challenge to those designing models of care delivery and financing is to provide good care to the homebound, to those who are most difficult to serve. I believe that no matter how the transformation proceeds, the frail and dependent will continue to have problems that require unique solutions. No organized system can account for the variety of circumstances found in an active home care practice where creative thinking will always have paramount value. It is also probable that many home care patients will remain near the residual cracks in any future system, with a tendency to fall through, and they will need home care physicians.

INFORMATION MANAGEMENT IN SYSTEMS

Earlier I briefly mentioned the importance of efficiently sharing clinical information. When physicians' offices are pressed to be fiscal resource managers, timely access to utilization data is doubly essential.

In Richmond managed care is growing fast but is not yet dominant. My physician group and hospital participate with dozens of payers. One sends me detailed utilization data. This IPA capitates and profiles primary care physicians while moving into specialty capitation. The utilization reports are instructive. I can see how much—and how little—various services actually cost. I have discovered surprising patterns among hospitals and consultants that then shape my future referrals. And I can better educate colleagues about cost-effectiveness.

It takes much work to move from an arrangement where providers and payers are all separate to a system where data are readily shared. Our hospital and our physician organization have separate information systems, which are now being linked. We will be able to give primary care physicians accurate internal utilization data, but we will still lack data about services provided outside our system. Some large systems accept the risk of being the payer and thereby obtain complete utilization data. Yet they too struggle with organizing data and giving information to providers in a useful format. Information has enormous value in practice management and in modifying physician behavior. However, surprisingly little administrative data now reach clinicians.

Information management is particularly vital in home care. These patients often have complex illnesses with long, relevant histories. They are seen by many providers, who do not directly communicate with each other very frequently. Patients develop new problems that cause them to move frequently between settings: home to physician office, emergency room, or hospital; hospital to rehabilitation unit; nursing home to home. Maintaining continuity is difficult. Yet one can picture a system of community-based care served by an indexed public database containing information about the availability and constraints of various service options, plus a shared clinical record that captures each patient's medical history, support systems, and providers.

Imagine the too familiar HCFA 485 form that authorizes home health care, the nurses' and therapists' visit notes, the home medical equipment orders, the physicians' progress notes, the recent hospital summary, and the current medication list, all consolidated. Everyone involved could know that home visits to CW must occur between 9 a.m. and 2 p.m., when the nurse's aide can open the door.

This is not an entirely futuristic vision. The Minimum Dataset for Long-Term Care[49] and the Medicare Uniform Clinical Dataset[50] are current examples of electronic clinical databases. Virginia has also developed a comprehensive Uniform Assessment Instrument, used by all agencies involved in long-term care; this followed the Virginia Long-Term Care Information System, used for the past 12 years. Another innovative private sector resource developed for home health nurses is a compact, hand-held minicomputer for capturing clinical data and generating reports. Home care software, including electronic clinical records, is proliferating wildly. Pittsburgh's Shadyside Hospital has an ambulatory clinical database, including hospital discharge data, readable from remote points with palm-top computers. There are also community resource databases, such as that developed at the Cincinnati Living-at-Home site. Several general considerations arise when contemplating this future.

First is technology. What makes this discussion more than an exercise in fantasy is remarkable progress with information handling. For instance, the "information superhighway" spans the globe, built on the Internet, which was first conceived merely 30 years ago. This overarching system of computers, cables, and satellites allows rapid long-distance data transport. Medical providers use such technology creatively. For example, a radiologist provides on-line service to three hospitals from his home, viewing transmitted video images of films and sending interpretations by modem.

Home care practice may run on local information roadways rather than superhighways, but the basic principles don't change. The telephone repairman recently came to my house. When he was finished, he plugged his hand-held keyboard into my phone jack and sent his entire service report to the company's computer. Cellular phones are also in common use. If we had the funds and the equipment, I could send clinical home care reports from my car between visits, including images such as electrocardiograms and X rays. If we were all connected by compatible systems, these data could be sent immediately to visiting nurses, physician consultants, or the emergency room. Yet few if any home care providers approach this level of sophistication, and there are several potential problems in implementing such a comprehensive information system.

Accuracy

One negative feature of rapid information sharing is the potential for distributing and perpetuating misinformation. I recently stopped in the emergency room to see IB, an office patient with severe ischemic heart disease. The intern asked about her recent pulmonary embolus, which surprised me because previous tests for pulmonary embolus were all conclusively negative. Yet topping the last hospital discharge sheet, entered by another physician, was the final diagnosis of pulmonary embolus. I was able to clarify the situation, but if this information had entered an electronic

network and been downloaded in several locations, a potentially dangerous misconception could have been disseminated and perpetuated. Data
are only as accurate as the person who enters them, and human data entry
errors are inevitable.

Quality Improvement

Jencks and Wilensky have proposed a new central data management
approach to quality improvement.[51] They cite research showing dramatic
regional variations in patterns and outcomes of care and variable effectiveness of physician review organizations. They espouse clinical practice
guidelines and suggest focusing quality improvement on common care
processes rather than unusual circumstances or mistakes. With the
Uniform Clinical Data Set, decision rules can identify cases for physician
review and provide large-scale measures of quality at institutions or in
localities. It will be interesting to see how this works. My experience with
the local physician review organization has been good: reviews have been
thorough, responsible, and clinically astute. However, I know of many
instances when suboptimal care was not reviewed, and I can see possible
value in a larger, systems approach. Computers can help, as long as they
are the servants and not the masters.

Kane discusses the difficulty in measuring the quality of long-term
care.[52] What does one measure? Longer life, cure rates, or normalized
blood pressures are quality benchmarks for other populations, but they
have less validity in long-term care, where care process and subjective
well-being are key parameters. Lately, quality monitoring in nursing
homes sometimes seems like a witch hunt rather than a constructive quality improvement process. Home care providers are more dispersed and
harder to study, but many of the same issues apply. Better methods are
clearly needed.

Data Sets

The Minimum Dataset for Long-Term Care, required in nursing homes,
is probably the best-known example of a centralized clinical database. It
contains demographic data, medical diagnoses, conditions and treatments,
functional status measures, mental status measures, and elements defining psychosocial well-being and relationships. Completing the dataset
requires about 90 minutes for a trained nurse and adds 30 minutes to a

new patient assessment. Defining the upper limits one encounters when many providers use such a system, trained observers achieved good inter-rater reliability coefficients, ranging from about 0.5 for mental status items to 0.8 for ADL dependencies, yet they were clearly far from perfect.[49] Reliability will be considerably lower in general use, especially during the early stages of the provider learning curve.

Confidentiality

One of the greatest concerns when embracing new information technology is privacy of patient information. Legitimate fear is expressed about the safety of CC, who is blind, elderly, and lives alone if it becomes known that she will leave her front door open after I call to plan a home visit. Highly sensitive information might similarly be exposed about diagnoses like mental illness, drug use, homosexuality, or AIDS; personal finances pertinent to qualifying for long-term care services; and other matters, whether sensitive or routine, that are the exclusive business of patients, their physicians, and those who govern resources. The paper system has leaks, but the electronic system is more dangerous. Can we achieve satisfactory security?

The problem of protecting sensitive information on computers has not yet been solved, but it is the subject of intensive work. Assuming that secure systems emerge, we still face the matter of patient acceptance. Patients are already hesitant about having sensitive information written in physicians' office charts, which are released only with patient approval. The anxiety may be far greater with shared computer records, particularly given the widely publicized ease with which "hackers" penetrate computer security.

Practicality of Disseminating Information Technology

Possibly the greatest barriers are issues of cost, chaos, and turf. Most physicians now bill electronically, and many use computerized appointment scheduling. A few even use computerized medical records. But although some physicians are facile with computers, most are moving slowly and reluctantly into the electronic era. Remember, too, physicians' well-known stubbornness and individuality.

The concept of "chaos" relates to the rich variety of computer hardware systems and software applications, which are often incompatible with each other. Perhaps the most familiar example is the gap separating personal computer users with IBM-compatible systems from those who use Macintosh systems. They can be forced to interface, but it is difficult. In Richmond my medical center is spending much money to link the computer system of our hospital with that of our physician organization. They are not very compatible. Moreover, the complex Baxter hospital system is not yet adapted to specific needs like those of MCV Home Care, so I maintain a D-Base database on a personal computer that can be easily shared only with other computers carrying D-Base software. It is easier to Xerox pages from the chart and send them by fax than it is to send electronic data. Furthering the challenge, our preferred home health agency partner uses Delta software. These examples illustrate the practical complexity of implementing the information systems that well-intended visionaries, myself included, may conceive.

Turf issues arise when competing providers are asked to share information, exemplified by the Cincinnati Living-at-Home site. Who would have control? Would the system carry patient data, resource information, or something else? Whose software and which type of hardware would be used? Who would have to reprogram? Would some agencies lose market share as a result of the linkage?

Finally, I mention cost. MCV Home Care recently received belated approval to rent three cellular phones. This required a letter of justification to the vice president for health sciences, and the request was approved mainly on the basis of provider safety in tough neighborhoods rather than of enhanced efficiency. The approval was embedded in a "right-sizing" effort at this public hospital beset by urban blight, recession-driven state budget cuts, increased competition and "cherry picking" in the private sector, and generalized efforts to constrain medical expenditures.

Contrast our situation with that of "free market" mobile services. Consider taxicabs, airport vans, or florists. Radio dispatch or telephone linkages are basic to mobile businesses. Computerized data transmission is the basis for credit card services, which are full of highly confidential personal information. These examples show that efficient communication is possible, given the necessary investment and the opportunity to recover the cost of new technologies by changing the prices of goods or services. These advances come slowly in medicine and may depend on serendipity or sponsorship.

Finally, as a colleague lamented when we encountered new inefficiencies after implementing a computerized office appointment scheduling system, computers usually provide more and better data, but they do not always save money.

REFERENCES

1. Kane RA, Kane TL. Systems of Long Term Care. In *Long Term Care: Principles, Programs, and Policies.* New York, NY: Springer Publishing Co; 1991; pp 306–309.
2. Ansak ML, Zawadski RT. On Lok CCODA: A Consolidated Model. In: Zawadski RT, ed. *Community-Based Systems of Long Term Care.* New York, NY: Haworth Press. 1984; pp 147–170.
3. Kane RL, Illston LH, Miller NA. Qualitative analysis of the Program of All-inclusive Care for the Elderly (PACE). *Gerontologist.* 1992; 32:771–780.
4. Newcomer R, Harrington C, Friedlob A. Social health maintenance organizations: Assessing their initial experience. *Health Serv Res.* 1990; 25:425–454.
5. Abrahams R, Von Sternberg T, Zeps D, Dunn S, Macko P. Integrating care for the geriatric patient: Examples from the social HMO (SHMO). *HMO Practice.* 1992; 6(4):12–19.
6. Manton KG, Newcomer R, Lowrimore GR, Vertrees JC, Harrington C. Social/health maintenance organization and fee-for-service health outcomes over time. *Health Care Financing Review.* 1993; 15(2): 173–202.
7. Remington L. Medicare HMO enrollment rising. *Remington Report.* April/May 1994; 32–33.
8. McMillan A. Trends in Medicare health maintenance organization enrollment: 1986–93. *Health Care Financing Review.* 1993; 15(1):135–146.
9. Kramer AM, Fox PD, Morgenstern N. Geriatric care approaches in health maintenance organizations. *J Am Geriatr Soc.* 1992; 40:1055–1067.
10. Fox HB, Wicks LB, Newacheck PW. State Medicaid health maintenance organization policies and special-needs children. *Health Care Financing Review.* 1993; 15(1):25–37.
11. Somers AR, Spears NL. *The Continuing Care Retirement Community: A Viable Option for Long Term Care?* New York, NY: Springer Publishing Co.; 1992.
12. Hall WJ, Griner PF. Cost-effective health care: The Rochester experience. *Health Affairs.* Spring 1993; 58–69.
13. Miles SH, Lurie N, Quam L, Caplan A. Health care reform in Minnesota. *N Engl J Med.* 1992; 327:1092–1095.
14. Kronick R, Goodman DC, Wennberg J. The marketplace in health care reform: The demographic limitations of managed competition. *N Engl J Med.* 1993; 328:148–152.

15. Stessman J, Ginsberg G, Hammerman-Rozenberg R, Friedman R, Roren D, Israeli A, Cohen A. Decreased hospital utilization by older adults attributable to a home hospitalization program. *J Am Geriatr Soc.* 1996; 44:59–598.

16. Bogdonoff MD, Hughes SL, Weissert WG, Paulsen E. *The Living-at-Home Program: Innovations in Service Access and Case Management.* New York, NY: Springer Publishing Co.; 1991.

17. Currie CT, Moore JT, Friedman SW, Warshaw GA. Assessment of elderly patients at home: A report of fifty cases. *J Am Geriatr Soc.* 1981; 29:398–401.

18. Hughes SL, Cordray DS, Spiker VA. Evaluation of a long-term care program. *Med Care.* 1984; 22:460–475.

19. Stein REK, Jessop DJ. Does pediatric home care make a difference for children with chronic illness? Findings from the Pediatric Ambulatory Care Treatment Study. *Pediatrics.* 1984; 73:845–853.

20. Scholtes P, Sherman J, Griffin M, Peterson C, Ryan J, Crosthwait N. Welcome Home: Management of medically fragile infants and children. *American Academy of Home Care Physicians Newsletter.* 1994; 6(2):13–14.

21. Galloway RF. House calls. *JAMA.* 1991; 266:786.

22. Reuler JB, Bax MJ, Sampson JH. Physician house call services for medically needy, inner-city residents. *Am J Public Health.* 1986; 76:1121–1134.

23. Spiegel AD. Home care: Doing right for the wrong reason. *NY State J Med.* 1993; 93(3):190–193.

24. Health and Policy Committee of the American College of Physicians. Home health care. *Ann Intern Med.* 1986; 105:454–460.

25. American Geriatrics Society Public Policy Committee. Home care and home care reimbursement. *J Am Geriatr Soc.* 1989; 37:1065–1066.

26. Brickner PH, Lam KL, Lee M, Lo W, Maja T, Wong A, Kellogg R. Caring for the Chinese homebound aged in New York City. *American Academy of Home Care Physicians Newsletter.* 1993; 5(2):16–17.

27. Miller RH. Containing use and expenditures in publicly insured long-term care programs. *Health Care Financing Review.* 1993; 14(4):181–207.

28. Clarfield AM, Bergman H. Medical home care services for the housebound elderly. *Can Med Assoc J.* 1991; 144:40–45.

29. Welch WP, Verrili MS, Katz SJ, Latimer E. A detailed comparison of physician services for the elderly in the United States and Canada. *JAMA.* 1996; 275:1410–1416.

30. ten Cate RS. Home visiting in the Netherlands. *J R Coll Gen Pract.* 1980; 30:347–353.

31. Jonsson A, Halldorsson T. Domiciliary assessment for geriatric patients in Reykjavik. *Gerontology.* 1981; 27:89–93.

32. Barker WH. *Adding Life to Years: Organized Geriatric Services in Great Britain and Implications for the United States.* Baltimore, Md: Johns Hopkins University Press; 1987.

33. Keenan JM, Boling PA, Schwartzberg JG, Olson L, Schneiderman M,

McCaffrey D, Ripsin CM. A national survey of the home visiting practice and attitudes of family physicians and internists. *Arch Intern Med.* 1992; 152:2025–2032.

34. Galinsky D, Schneiderman K, Lowenthal MN. *Isr J Med Sci.* 1983; 19: 841–844.

35. Berg S, Branch LG, Doyle AE, Sundstrom G. Institutional and home-based long-term care alternatives: The 1965–1985 Swedish experience. *Gerontologist.* 1988; 28:825–829.

36. Melin AL, Hakansson S, Bygren LO. The cost-effectiveness of rehabilitation in the home: A study of Swedish elderly. *Am J Public Health.* 1993; 83: 356–361.

37. Della Penna RD. A model long term care program using geriatricians and geriatric nurses practitioners in an HMO. Presented at the annual meeting of the American Geriatric Society, May 19, 1994, Los Angeles, Calif.

38. Thomas K, Birch S, Milner P, Nicholl J, Westlake L, Williams B. Estimates of general practitioner workload: A review. *J R Coll Gen Pract.* 1989; 39:509–513.

39. Hallam L, Metcalfe DHH. Seasonal variations in the process of care in urban general practice. *J Epidemiol Community Health.* 1985; 39:90–93.

40. Bucquet D, Jarman B, White P. Factors associated with home visiting in an inner London general practice. *Br Med J.* 1985; 290:1480–1483.

41. Lawhorne LW, Walker G, Zweig SC, Snyder J. Who cares for Missouri's Medicaid nursing home residents? Characteristics of attending physicians. *J Am Geriatr Soc.* 1993; 41:454–458.

42. Schueler MS, Harris DL, Goodenough GK, Collette L. House calls in Utah. *West J Med.* 1987; 147(1):92–94.

43. Leutz W, Malone J, Kistner M, O'Bar T, Ripley JM, Sandhaus M. Financial performance in the social health maintenance organization, 1985–88. *Health Care Financing Review.* 1990; 12(1):9–18.

44. Inouye SK, Wagner DR, Acampora D, Horwitz RI, Cooney LM, Hurst LD, Tinetti ME. A predictive index for functional decline in hospitalized elderly medical patients. *J Gen Intern Med.* 1993; 8:645–652.

45. Fishman LM, Emro MA. Active Use of Serial Functional Assessment Improves Outcome and Shortens Acute Geriatric Hospitalization. *Top Geriatr Rehabil.* 1994; 9(3):16–29.

46. Solomon DH, Wagner DR, Marenberg ME, Acampora D, Cooney LM, Inouye SK. Predictors of formal home health use in elderly patients after hospitalization. *J Am Geriatr Soc.* 1993; 41:961–966.

47. Jackson ME, Eichorn A, Sokoloff S, Van Tassel J. Evaluating the predictive validity of nursing home pre-admission screens. *Health Care Financing Review.* 1993; 14(4):169–180.

48. Capitman JA. Community-based long-term care models, target groups, and impacts on service use. *Gerontologist.* 1986; 26:389–397.

49. Morris JN, Hawes C, Fries BE, Phillips CD, Mor V, Katz S, Murphy K, Drugovich ML, Friedlob AS. Designing the National Resident Assessment Instrument for Nursing Homes. *Gerontologist.* 1990; 30:293–306.

50. Audet AM, Scott D. The Uniform Clinical Data Set: An evaluation of the proposed national database for Medicare's quality review program. *Ann Intern Med.* 1993; 119:1209–1213.

51. Jencks SF, Wilensky GR. The health care quality improvement initiative: A new approach to quality assurance in Medicare. *JAMA.* 1992; 268:900–903.

52. Kane RL. Improving the quality of long-term care. *JAMA.* 1995; 273: 1376–1380.

PART *III*

Home Health Care in Our Society

CHAPTER 9

Present and Projected Demands for Home Health

E arlier chapters have discussed approaches to care of the frail and immobile. I now turn to health policy, financing, and service delivery capacity. To know how many physicians, nurse practitioners, and physician assistants will be needed for home care and how their time will be spent, one must rely on clinical epidemiology and population-wide estimates of functional dependency, using well-established research techniques. Here is the bottom line: about 2 million people are chronically homebound due to functional impairment. This group will grow to 3 million by the year 2020, with two-thirds being elderly and 1 million 85 or older.

It is well known that the elderly are an important group when planning for health care delivery, as reviewed by Beck and Ouslander.[1] In 1979 the elderly were 11% of the population, yet they accounted for 30% of health care spending. They used one-third of acute care beds, 90% of nursing home beds, and over one-fourth of prescription drugs. Life expectancy increased from 47 years in 1900 to 72 years in 1975, and it is now near 80. With the baby boom, component, the population aged 65 and over will double from 23 million in 1982 to 50 million in 2030. The number of those over age 85 will increase fourfold, and this group will use home care extensively. Factors other than age also create important subgroups needing home care; minorities, for example, have poorer health and fewer resources.

When planning for the future, definitions of health and health care are very important. For example, the 1982 WHO goals for health care of the elderly were broad: "Keep the elderly in good health and happiness in their own houses for as long as possible." Lack of health can further be defined in many ways: as disease, as illness, as loss of function, or loss of social relevance. And the elderly may perceive health and need differently from their evaluators and caregivers. In home care the boundaries of medical need and those separating patient need from caregiver need require constant attention lest social issues overwhelm providers. We can no longer afford to define health too broadly. Finally, when looking at the total population, we must again realize that home care is far from being a geriatric field. Nearly half of community dwellers with severe functional impairment are under age 65.

WHO WILL NEED HOME HEALTH CARE?

The answer depends on how we organize care. If I continue practicing till age 66, in the year 2020, will I visit frail patients only in nursing homes, senior apartment complexes, and life care communities? Or will many still live in private homes with overextended, undertrained informal caregivers? Will an advanced transportation system bring these people to a community center? Will I sit in a conference room directing a team of professionals who give home care or provide consultation by video-telephone while I myself am rarely in the field? When patients need help, will society give help? As you read, picture your own community and think of your neighbors. Where are the homebound? How many are there now, and how will things change in 20 years' time?

The best data on the numbers of chronologically homebound people come from national surveys of need and service utilization. Yet the best data are imperfect. Key items like functional status are measured differently from study to study.[2,3] Crucial facts about the local environment, informal supports, and their relationship to outcomes are impossible to capture. Some of the most needy, such as the "shut-ins" and the oldest old, are hard to find and count.

Still, with national data we can construct predictive mathematical models. For example, why do people put relatives in nursing homes? Risk factors are known,[4] and Weissert developed a multivariate model with 18 variables that correctly predicted nursing home residence 98% of the time.[5] The following variables are listed in order of weight:

1. Toileting/feeding dependency
2. Bathing/dressing dependency
3. Mental disorder
4. Cancer, anemia, kidney trouble, and/or digestive disease
5. Circulatory disease
6. Not married
7. White (caucasian) race
8. Poverty
9. Nervous system disease
10. Injury
11. Diabetes
12. Respiratory disease
13. Arthritis/rheumatism
14. Mobility dependency
15. Male sex
16. Age (older)
17. Vacant nursing home beds in the community
18. Hot climate

Yet models have limits. This one would identify the elderly, diabetic, widowed MM as someone at high risk of institutionalization. She might be targeted by a program to prevent nursing home placement. We would then find that her family stood by her in an overheated lower-middle-income home for years, despite strokes, bedfast dependency, bedsores, dementia, incontinence, and hourlong, painstaking oral feedings. After all that, it was the loss of speech and the shock of needing to give gastrostomy feedings after her latest stroke that caused institutionalization. Ironically, her care was really simplified by the gastrostomy. Then, the shock dissipated, a new bedsore alarmed the family, a feeding schedule compatible with their work hours was designed, and MM came back home. No model could predict this sequence. Worse yet, models lose accuracy as patient characteristics diverge from the highest-risk profiles. Models help with large-scale planning, but finally, individuals must manage individual cases. When one gives care in the real world, the best-laid plans meet unexpected obstacles.

TABLE 9.1 U.S. Population in Millions

Year	Total population	65–74 Years	75–84 Years	85 Years and over	65 Years and over
1990	250	18	10	3	32
2020	296	30	14	7	51
2050	309	30	21	16	67

A LOOK AT SOME BASIC DEMOGRAPHICS

It is common knowledge that there will be a striking increase in senior citizens as the baby boomers age. Table 9.1 shows projections from 1980 census data, adapted from Gilford.[6] The picture hasn't changed much since 1980.

Two key issues arise from these data. A fairly constant, substantial number of young people will continue using home care, and the disproportionate increase in elders will bring many with serious new functional limitations. Preventive strategies may blunt the impact, but this is a tidal wave that will arrive no matter how actively we pursue prevention or biotechnical intervention. Frail elders, many already underserved, will double or triple in number. Second, the ratio of elders needing care to younger adults able to give care will rise sharply. The total population will increase by only 20% while frail elders double or even triple. Meanwhile, more and younger women are entering the work force. We will need more caregiving, and we will have fewer traditional caregivers.

The younger people needing home care fall more easily into groups. Care of people with AIDS is increasingly given in outpatient settings, homes, and hospices. Comparing 1991 with 1983, AIDS deaths occurred in hospitals far less often: 57% of deaths compared with 92%.[7] In 1988, 21% of AIDS deaths occurred outside hospitals. Of those 4,317 deaths, 85% occurred at home. Only 13% were in hospices or nursing homes. The Centers for Disease Control estimated the prevalence of HIV infection at 700,000 cases in 1996.[8] It is hard to predict society's response to this epidemic, such as expanding hospices and nursing homes. Still, the cost of AIDS is great,[9] with correspondingly rapid growth of AIDS home care.

Another group needing home care is the seriously ill children kept alive by advanced technology. Vladeck[10] finds between 10,000 and 30,000 "technology dependent" children among the 400,000 children with three or more ADL limitations. Medicaid payments for home health services to 561,319 patients under age 21 totaled $2.9 billion in 1992, or $5,000 per recipient.[11] This was more than half of the $4.9 billion spent by Medicaid on home health for nonelderly persons. Such children use a great deal of home care.

A third group is composed of young and middle-aged adults who are born with neurological deficits, suffer traumatic injury to the brain or spinal cord, or develop degenerative neuromuscular disorders such as polio, multiple sclerosis, myotonic dystrophy, or amyotrophic lateral sclerosis. They usually remain impaired for life. Spinal cord injury affected about 200,000 persons in the mid-1980s, with a mean age of 31 and a long life expectancy.[12] Some younger adults with neuromuscular impairment become remarkably self-sufficient, but many require extensive long-term help. Mental retardation also produces ADL or IADL limitations in nearly 1 million people aged 18 to 65, of whom only a quarter live in institutions. Thus, 475,000 nonelderly adults have disabilities causing dependence in three or more ADLs.[10]

Fourth are the psychiatrically impaired. Among the nonelderly with serious mental illness, 3.4 of 3.6 million live in the community rather than in institutions. Of these, 750,000 need help with ADLs or IADLs.[10] The elderly demented population whose incapacity derives mainly from cognitive impairment is hard to measure because of the overlap between Alzheimer's disease, other dementias, and physical illness. Dementia has a reported prevalence of 3% to 5% in those over 64 and as high as 28% among those over 84.[13] Many psychiatrically impaired people need home care.

CAN WE FORESTALL FRAILTY AND DEPENDENCY BY BETTER CARE?

Our society has made advances in both preventive care and medical treatment. Deaths from coronary disease and stroke are declining. Life expectancy at birth is over 72 years for men and 78 years for women. Life expectancy for those reaching age 65 is about 15 years for men and nearly 20 years for women. Those who reach 85 live another 5 years.

Accordingly, Fries[14] and others talk of compressing morbidity, the idea that people can enjoy good health until late in life, then rapidly decline and die as they approach the natural life span of homo sapiens. This is an optimistic vision, in which medical advances square the morbidity curve (see Figure 9.1).

This concept has been critiqued. One issue is practicality; it is doubtful that we can fully realize the promise of medical advances. So just as death and taxes remain certain, chronic illnesses like arthritis, cardiovascular disease, dementia, and cancer will likely still take their toll. Also, the more people we keep alive till late in life, the more the overall burden of illness will accumulate population-wide. Misery may be experienced for a smaller fraction of each person's longer life, but there will still be a descending shoulder at the end of the population's active life expectancy curve. The area under that curve will increase, and in that zone will lie the work of many home care physicians. This difference between total life expectancy and active life expectancy is shown in Figure 9.2.

HOME CARE FOR THOSE WHO ARE *NOT* CHRONICALLY HOMEBOUND

As we analyze how many persons will need physician home care, we shouldn't neglect those with home care needs who are not under the right-hand shoulder of Fries's curve. Sometimes home care is simply a less expensive, more pleasant alternative to institutional care. Examples are socially active full-time workers on home dialysis or businessmen taking home intravenous antibiotics for osteomyelitis. These options are increasing as home care technology improves.

Another large and important group of low-intensity home care patients are those with specific, limited, and often simple needs, such as a walker, a new light in the hall, a handrail by the toilet, or an emergency call system. My 96-year-old patient ET unavoidably fell and broke her hip. Her call button then proved vital. The public health model, typified by community-based influenza vaccination campaigns, also uses mobile care to prevent serious illness. This patient group is more relatively mobile and less homebound. The home care intervention is made to prevent morbid complications or to further improve function and quality of life. These patients are hard to count, but they number in the tens of millions.

In a more radical view, home care might even be used by people who are basically healthy, exemplified by video consultation with physicians.

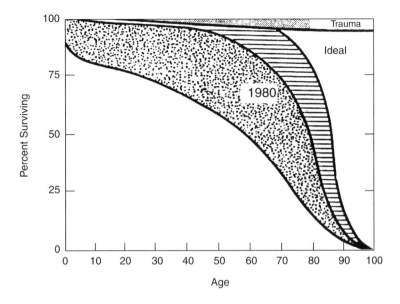

Figure 9.1 The increasingly rectangular survival curve. About 80% (stippled area) of the difference between the 1900 curve and the ideal curve (stippled area plus hatched area) had been eliminated by 1980. Trauma is now the dominant cause of death in early life.

Telephone medicine, now commonplace in medical practice, may be an early manifestation of that future. The potential demand for home care by nonhomebound patients is enormous. However, in the near future most of home care will still be used by people who are homebound, temporarily or chronically, and who need much help. The next big question is to define what makes people homebound and to estimate their needs for professional home care.

DEFINING HOMEBOUND

Branch et al. write: "Barriers to access and utilization of health services among the populace are reasoned to be not only financial but also psychological, informational, social, organizational, spatial, and temporal."[15] They mathematically model use of physician visits, hospital days, home care, and dental care. Yet the models explain only a small portion of the

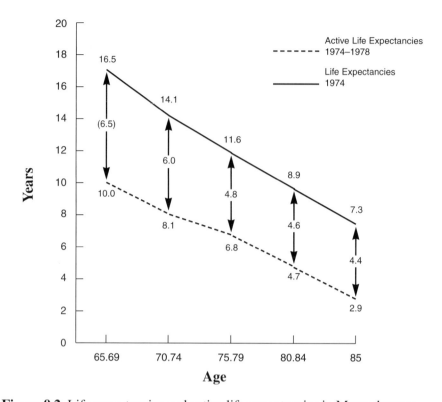

Figure 9.2 Life expectancies and active life expectancies in Massachusetts.

Reprinted with permission from *Health Status and the Quality of Life*. Copyright © 1988 by the National Academy of Sciences. Courtesy of the National Academy Press, Washington, D.C.

variance in service use, perhaps because health care is an individualized phenomenon. To a clinician, the definition of homebound is indeed imprecise. I may ask: Overall, how difficult or costly is it for this patient to reach the office? What creates the barrier to getting medical care, and how can it best be overcome? This requires judgment, experience, and case-by-case choices.

For example, one old woman with three complete ADL limitations and several serious medical conditions lives with a muscular, devoted son. She comes to the office regularly in her wheelchair and enjoys the opportunity to leave home. Another woman with virtually identical medical and physical problems lives with a little old man, "Pops," who has limited capability, in a small house with eight front steps. She cannot easily leave home. Such are the details that dictate the need for physician home care. As Branch noted, being homebound is a complex phenomenon. Following are some case examples.

DS is a young man with amyotrophic lateral sclerosis (Lou Gehrig's disease). He can't move any part of his body except his head, and he is on continuous mechanical home ventilation. Transporting DS for routine medical care makes no sense.

WW is a large man, paralyzed on one side from a stroke. He lives on the second floor of his house with his wife, lives in his bed, and travels only by ambulance. It is an ordeal for the family, patient, and ambulance crew to carry WW downstairs, up to the clinic, and back home. The trip costs over $300 and can't be easily arranged except in emergencies. WW is chronically, totally homebound.

AC is a young, partially quadriplegic man. He has some use of his arms and can come to the office in a wheelchair if his friend is around and the old pickup truck works. When his friend is out or the truck breaks down, new medical complaints create home care needs.

LH is a blind diabetic woman with poor circulation in her legs that limits her to walking short distances. Her son works days, but given advance notice he can take her to some doctors' visits. A mental health outreach worker who followed LH at home for depression called to say she could no longer afford the time to bring LH to my office. I put LH on the "nonurgent" house call list. Then the worker called again. LH had cut her leg. I saw her at home the next day, treating a potentially dangerous infection that LH could not see or feel.

VS was born at 24 weeks and developed bronchopulmonary dysplasia, requiring long-term ventilator care. After a year of institutional care, a home care plan was developed by her HMO, her primary pediatrician, a pulmonologist, and several other home care professionals. The family managed 2 years of home care at an estimated savings of $1 million. The small child and ventilator were relatively portable compared with an adult, but transportation was still hard, and physician house calls were highly valued.

These cases should convey the many dimensions that contribute to being homebound. Patients report being so devastated by the rigors of visits to outpatient settings that it takes days to recover. Caregivers miss work or must pay for child care when they accompany patients to appointments. Whether homebound status derives from such personal concerns or the dollar cost of transportation, the constellation of elements is such that the burdens of seeking conventional care exceed the burdens of delivering home care.

Some of these considerations are the basis for administrative definitions of homebound. Medicare regulates home health care, using a specific definition of homebound as one essential criterion. A portion of the regulation reads: "An individual does not have to be bedridden to be considered as confined to his home. However, the condition of these patients should be such that there exists a normal inability to leave the home and, consequently, leaving their homes would require a considerable and taxing effort." A person can be homebound and still leave home for medical treatment, day care, dialysis, and chemotherapy or radiation therapy. Occasional trips for nonmedical reasons fall within the framework as long as they are infrequent. Illness or injury that result in the need for supportive devices for mobility (crutches, canes, wheelchairs, walkers) or special transportation constitute homebound status, as does serious psychiatric illness.

State Medicaid programs offer minor variations on this theme. Virginia defines "essentially homebound" to include people who need assistance from others or use special equipment to leave home; who have mental or emotional problems that cause them to refuse to leave home or that make it unsafe for them to leave home unattended, who are ordered by physicians to restrict activity due to a weakened condition (e.g., following surgery or heart disease), or who have active communicable diseases. Virginia Medicaid also approves home care if the combined cost of transportation plus treatment exceeds the cost of home care, if the patient is unreliable in seeking physician care and would have to be admitted to a hospital or nursing home because of missing treatment, if visits are for instruction to the patient in situations where this can better be accomplished at home, or if the duration of treatment is such that rendering it outside the home is impractical.

Other "objective" definitions of *homebound* have been tried. One author defined as homebound those who answered the question "About how often do you get out of your house/building for any reason?" with "Never or almost never except for emergencies."[16] Compared with direct clinician evaluation, this definition performed poorly. Being able to go out is not the same as going out.

Homebound status is individualized in daily clinical reality, but planning budgets and defining policies at a societal level does not permit using case-by-case formulations. Standard methods must be used to predict demand and define coverage. Physical dysfunction is the main proxy used for potential home care need, and large epidemiologic surveys are the mainstay for home care policy.

TABLE 9.2 Persons with Dependency Characteristic (Million)

	Total dependents	Personal care dependents	Mobility dependents
Total	4.9	2.9	2.0
Under 65	1.6	0.8	0.8
Over 65	3.3	2.1	1.2
Female	3.2	1.8	1.4
Male	1.7	1.0	0.7

TABLE 9.3 Living Situation

	Community (millions)	Nursing home (millions)
Personal care		
Need help bathing/dressing	1.1	0.4
Need help toileting/eating	0.7	0.7
Mobility		
Need help outside house	1.7	0.05
Need help inside house	0.2	0.01

TABLE 9.4 Community Dwellers (Thousands, % of Population Subset)

	Dependent total	Dependent for personal care	Dependent for mobility
Total	5,444 (2.6)	1,877 (0.9)	775 (0.4)
Under age 65	2,626 (1.4)	820 (0.5)	240 (0.1)
Age 65 and over	2,829 (11.7)	1,057 (4.4)	535 (2.2)
Age 65–74	1,064 (7.1)	345 (2.3)	196 (1.3)
Age 75 and over	1,765 (20.6)	712 (8.4)	339 (4.0)

Tables 9.2–9.4 are from "Estimating the Long-Term Care Population Prevalence Rate & Selected Characteristics, " by W.G. Weissert, 1985, *Health Care Financing Review 6* (4), 83–91. Reprinted with permission of Health Care Financing Administration.

**TABLE 9.5 Older Persons with Dependency Characteristic
(Thousands) Projected for Year 2000**

Age group	Total	Institutionalized	Dependent for personal care	Otherwise dependent
Total	6,330	2,367	1,889	2,074
65–69	547	89	172	286
70–74	839	179	237	423
75–79	1,197	324	359	514
80–84	1,163	488	504	171
≥85	2,584	1,287	617	680

POPULATION-BASED STUDIES OF DEPENDENCY AND HOME CARE NEED

Weissert described long-term care using combined data from the National Health Interview Survey (NHIS; 1977, 1979, 1980), the census (1980), and the National Nursing Home Survey (1977).[17] The National Health Interview Survey studied over 100,000 people on each wave, 11% aged 65 and over. Long-term care was defined, excluding people with psychiatric incapacity:

> The long-term care population consists of all persons, regardless of age or diagnosis, who, because of a chronic condition, require or receive human help in personal care, mobility, household activities, or home-administered health care services. Personal care includes eating, continence, transferring (e.g. moving from bed to chair, or bed to floor), toileting, dressing, and bathing. Mobility includes walking and going outside. Household activities include meal preparation, money management, shopping and chores, excluding yard work. Home-administered health services include injections, dressings, physical therapy, and other health care services.

In the study, dependency was partitioned into two categories: "personal care" (human help with bathing, dressing, toileting, eating) and "mobility" (assistance getting around inside or outside). See Tables 9.2, 9.3, 9.4, and 9.5.

Thus, we see that the community-dwelling long-term care population is larger than the nursing home population. And though dependency increases rapidly after age 65, the total number of functionally dependent younger people is large. Clearly, the projected changes are dramatic, and the type of dependency also matters greatly. Of those dependent in toileting and eating, 51% were in nursing homes, compared with 29% of those dependent in bathing and dressing and only 3% of those with reduced mobility inside or outside of the house.

The comparison of nursing home long-term care and community long-term care begs a digression. Nursing homes have been the focus of long-term care reform, partly because the population is "visible" and partly because it is easier to study. Visiting a nursing home, one notices the high degree of dependency: bathing (90%), dressing (80%), toileting (60%), continence (50%), and eating (40%).[18] It is hard to picture these patients at home until you have seen hundreds of such cases, as I have.

As a group, community dwellers have a wider range of functionality. The most severely debilitated subset is about the same size as the most dependent nursing home subset or perhaps slightly smaller, but the total home care population is much, much larger than the nursing home population. Thus, it is interesting to see Vladeck's 1993 estimate that $75 billion was spent on institutional care, whereas only $33 billion was spent on community care. Of the $33 billion, Medicare paid $9 billion, and Medicaid paid $6 billion. Private sources paid almost half. Informal caregivers, people I see in homes all over Richmond, carry the thankless load that covers the difference between nursing home and home care spending.

Experienced home care providers will also substantiate the enormous importance of social issues in home care. Poverty and dysfunctional social supports complicate home care in ways that those without experience have difficulty appreciating. To measure the social dimension, Elston used the 1984 NHIS Supplement on Aging and the 1986 Area Health Resources File System to predict local populations with dependency.[19] Basic NHIS data showed that about 2.0 million of elderly community dwellers had one or more ADL dependencies, whereas 4.2 million others had only IADL dependencies. The study added factors like physician availability, nursing home and hospital beds, population density, climate, and poverty to models that predicted limited function. Dependency increased with age, non-Caucasian race, size of the local geriatric population, and poverty. After adjusting for other factors, ADL dependency increased dramatically with poverty, doubling from low-poverty to high-poverty localities. We must include such factors when planning for the future.

TABLE 9.6 Highest Level of Disability

Disability level	Persons (millions)	% of all elderly
Nondisabled	23.9	77.4
IADLs only	1.4	4.4
1–2 ADLs	2.0	6.5
3–4 ADLs	1.1	3.5
5–6 ADLs	0.8	2.7
Institutionalized	1.7	5.5
Total	**30.8**	**100.0**

Adapted from "Estimates of Change in Chronic Disability and Institutional Incidence and Prevalence Rates in the U.S. Elderly Population from the 1982, 1984, and 1989 National Long Term Care Survey," by Manton et al., 1993, *Journal of Gerontology*, p.5159, Copyright © 1993, The Gerontological Society of America. Adapted with permission.

We must also understand how needs change with time's passage. The Established Populations for Epidemiologic Studies of the Elderly (EPESE) project studied over 10,000 community-dwelling elderly from three areas: rural Iowa; East Boston, Massachusetts; and New Haven, Connecticut.[20] This study showed that between 2% and 6% of elderly community dwellers have serious trouble with basic mobility at some point during each year. Data for those aged 85 and above are less precise due to small sample sizes. Branch et al. then followed one EPESE population for 2 years in East Boston,[21] a geographically defined community. They tracked people newly entering a medical home care program in which a team of physicians, nurse practitioners, nurses, social workers, physical therapists, and aides managed care at home. New use of home care was 12 times more likely by those aged 85 and above, than by those aged 65 to 74. After adjusting for age and sex, the rate of new home care use was 3.2% in 2 years.

This study brings the dimension of time to cross-sectional studies of functional status and home care. It also blends several types of home care and does not specifically distinguish the physician component. Still, extrapolating, if the elderly were 15% of 250 million people, or 37 million, then 600,000 would *newly* use such an interdisciplinary service each year, assuming a community structured and populated like East Boston. This estimate is probably low. Providers other than the East Boston team delivered home care in the area, and unrecognized or unmet needs are not counted. Finally, this was an incidence study. The number of home care users at any one time would be higher because of chronic (prevalent) cases. Regardless, 600,000 of these patients per year would be a huge load.

Two other national surveys consolidate the functional deficit story. The 1980 Medical Care Utilization and Expenditure Survey found about 5.5 million people with two or more ADL limitations. Of these, 2.3 million were age 65 and over, and 132,000 were under age 19.[22] Then the National Long Term Care Survey, conducted in 1982, 1984, and 1989, defined chronic disability as inability, lasting (or expected to last) 90 days or more, to perform an ADL without personal assistance or equipment or an IADL because of a disability or health problem (including "old age"). Data from 1989 are shown in Table 9.6.[23]

People with three or more ADL deficits usually have difficulty moving around, including going to see physicians. And as any office-based physician can attest, even the more mobile patients with major ADL deficits require extra time and attention. Wiener found about 800,000 community-dwelling elders needing human help to transfer from bed to chair or use the toilet.[2] Office practice is difficult with these patients.

Taking the next step and linking functional deficits to home care eligibility is the focus of an excellent study by Stone and Murtaugh, again using the 1984 National Long Term Care Survey.[24] Functional deficits are defined as requiring human assistance to perform specific activities for at least three months. A patient who gets to the bathroom alone using only a walker would be independent for toileting. Five ADLs are analyzed: eating, transferring in and out of bed, toileting, bathing, and dressing. The IADLs studied include meal preparation, taking medication, telephoning, doing laundry, getting around outside, grocery shopping, and money management. Table 9.7 shows the estimated number of elders with ADL deficits, including 471,000 who need active help to get out of bed.

Table 9.8 then shows how the degree of impairment affects the number of people who might use home care, depending on eligibility criteria. Note the large number of community-dwelling elders with three or more ADL deficits, and imagine how life is for them. The 536,000 who require active help for three or more ADLs are 2% of the community-dwelling elderly, the 1.3 million needing active or standby help with 2 ADLs are 6.1%, and the 4.1 million who need some help with any ADL or IADL are 15.5%.

Varying eligibility criteria create a huge range in the number of people who might use home care. Limiting eligibility to those with only year-round incapacity diminishes potential users by about a third. The most restrictive parameters were 3 or more ADL deficits requiring active human help and lasting at least 12 months. These defined a population of 411,000.

TABEL 9.7 Number of Noninstitutionalized Elderly Individuals Who Meet Alternative Disability Criteria by Type of Help Required

	Type of help required			
	Active		Active or standby	
Disability criterion	Number (thousand)	Percentage of noninstitutionalized elders in U.S.	Number (thousands)	Percentage of noninstitutionalized elders in U.S.
Three or more ADLs	536 (±50)	2.0	984 (±66)	3.7
Two or more ADLs	857 (±62)	3.2	1,350 (±74)	5.1
Any ADL	1,564 (±78)	5.9	2,064 (±84)	7.8
Any ADL or daily IADL*	2,474 (±87)	9.3	2,737 (±88)	10.3
Any ADL or IADL	4,048 (±84)	15.2	4,124 (±83)	15.5

Note. The 95% confidence interval is calculated by adding and subtracting the number in parentheses. Source: 1984 National Long-Term Care Survey.

* Daily IADLs are meal preparation, taking medication, and telephoning.

TABLE 9.8 Number of Noninstitutionalized Elderly Individuals Meeting Alternative Disability Criteria including a Duration Requirement (Number in Thousands)

Disability criterion	Duration requirement					
	3+ months		6+ months		12+ months	
Active help						
Three or more ADLs	536	(±50)	485	(±48)	411	(±45)
Two or more ADLs	857	(±62)	772	(±59)	670	(±56)
Any ADL	1,564	(±78)	1,405	(±75)	1,232	(±72)
Any ADL or daily IADL*	2,474	(±87)	2,318	(±86)	2,137	(±85)
Any ADL or IADL	4,048	(±84)	3,871	(±85)	3,604	(±87)
Active or standby help						
Three or more ADLs	984	(±66)	882	(±63)	745	(±58)
Two or more ADLs	1,350	(±74)	1,208	(±71)	1,049	(±67)
Any ADL	2,064	(±84)	1,862	(±82)	1,634	(±79)
Any ADL or daily IADL*	2,737	(±88)	2,556	(±88)	2,355	(±87)
Any ADL or IADL	4,124	(±83)	3,938	(±85)	3,671	(±87)

Note. The 95% confidence interval is calculated by adding and subtracting the number in parentheses. Source: 1984 National Long-Term Care Survey.

* Daily IADLs are meal preparation, taking medication, and telephoning.

Using the least restrictive criteria (any ADL or IADL deficit requiring either active or standby assistance and lasting as little as 3 months), those eligible for home care would number 4.1 million. The middle ground is defined by people with two ADL deficits, numbering 875,000 if the criterion is "needing active human help" or 1.3 million if we include those who need only standby help. Remember that these data reflect only the elderly. An equally large number of people with similar levels of impairment are now found among those under age 65, bringing the total current middle ground to somewhere around 2 million persons.

The size of the home care–eligible population is critical to health care funders. Doubling the number of eligible persons might double the cost, now measured in tens of billions.[3,25] Home care use seems to be controlled by demand rather than by supply,[26] though recent findings or dramatic regional differences have raised some questions on this point.[27] As a home care physician, I see the situation differently from an administrator picturing a financial drain with each added eligibility criterion. Lacking vested financial interests yet being interested in outcomes and efficiency, I would expect the more functional members of Stone and Murtaugh's 4.1 million to visit doctors' offices. Most of them would need only occasional, inexpensive home care, such as grab bars, walkers, and short-term therapy. They might also need transportation and improved living options.

On the other hand, most of those in the severely impaired 411,000 are completely and chronically homebound, needing many formal and informal services, including house calls. Even for them, physician and professional provider involvement in home care would be graduated, being most intensive for those most medically unstable. Likewise, the middle ground cohort, numbering about 1 million, impaired to the point of requiring human help with two of five basic ADLs, would often benefit from some direct physician home care.

Finally, the NHIS shows what happens as populations age. In the 1984 survey, 594 of 1,791 persons aged 80 and over were physically "able." Fewer than half were still "able" 2 years later, but only 10% had died.[28] Thus, many became dependent. The EPESE subjects showed a similar pattern after 2 years.[29] Primary care physicians know that when one follows older individuals longitudinally in a practice, many become infirm and need more help. Because is difficult to predict which individuals will decline, flexible, continuous delivery systems are paramount, and established physicians' practice profiles will differ from those of newcomers.

CLOSING THOUGHTS

Vladeck recently synthesized data from several sources with other issues related to use of community long-term care.[10] The authors report that 42.6 million people (16% of U.S. citizens) have physical or mental disabilities, and 12.6 million use long-term care, defined as assistance with ADLs or IADLs. Forty-two percent are under age 65. There are 500,000 children, 4.8 million nonelderly adults, and 7.3 million elderly. Community dwelling is the rule, representing 10.3 million of the 12.6 million. Among the 12.6 million are 400,000 children and 475,000 young adults with three or more ADL dependencies. If one adds the 750,000 elderly with three or more ADL deficits in the National Long-Term Care Survey, the total is 1.6 million people, a conservative estimate of current chronic home care need.

The future will be much different because of the "graying of America." The million people I dubbed Stone's middle ground represent 3% to 5% of the noninstitutionalized elderly. Unless institutionalization becomes more common, this middle ground will expand to nearly 2 million by the time I am considering retirement. Moreover, those 85 and above, of whom 20% have serious immobility, will have doubled, constituting a million homebound. The younger immobile population should remain fairly constant, so the total number of homebound people may near 3 million.

Now, consider your own community. Based on these studies, I suspect that about 1% of the elderly living in my Richmond, Virginia, community are homebound by almost any definition. The urban area holds 750,000 people. About 15% are elderly. This means approximately 1,000 are elderly homebound, with a similar number of younger adults and children who are comparably immobile bringing the total to 2,000. Beyond these severely incapacitated people, another 2% to 5% of the seniors have significant functional deficits. Many of them need periodic skilled home care, including house calls and physician care management. Adding nongeriatric cases brings this needy population to 10,000, beside which my home care team and its 150 patients seems very small. This thought introduces the subject for chapter 10: How to meet the need.

REFERENCES

1. Ouslander JG, Beck JC. Defining the health problems of the elderly. *Ann Rev Public Health.* 1982; 3:55–83.1982.

2. Wiener JM, Hanley RJ, Clark R, Van Nostrand JF. Measuring activities of daily living: Comparisons across national surveys. *J Gerontol.* 1990; 45(6):S229–237.

3. Kunkel SR, Applebaum RA. Estimating the prevalence of long-term disability for an aging society. *J Gerontol.* 1992; 47(5):S253–S260.

4. Shapiro E, Tate R. Who is really at risk of institutionalization? *Gerontologist.* 1988; 28:237–245.

5. Weissert WG, Cready CM. Toward a model for improved targeting of aged at risk of institutionalization. *Health Serv Res.* 1989; 24:485–510.

6. Social, Economic, and Demographic Changes Among the Elderly. In: Guilford, DM, ed, *The Aging Population in the Twenty-First Century.* Washington, DC: National Academy Press, 1988, p. 54.

7. Kelly JJ, Chu SY, Buehler JW, et al. AIDS deaths shift from hospital to home. *Am J Public Health.* 1993; 83:1433–1437.

8. Holmberg SD. The estimated prevalence and incidence of HIV in 96 large US metropolitan areas. *Am J Public Health.* 1996; 85(6):647–654.

9. Hellinger FJ. The lifetime cost of treating a person with HIV. *JAMA.* 1993; 270:474–478.

10. Vladeck BC, Miller NA, Clauser SB. The changing face of long term care. *Health Care Financing Review.* 1993; 14(4):5–23.

11. *Statistical Report on Medical Care: Eligibles, Recipients, Payments, and Services.* Washington, DC: Health Care Financing Administration, Bureau of Data Management and Strategy. HCFA Report 2082.

12. Ditunno JF, Formal CS. Chronic spinal cord injury. *N Engl J Med.* 1994; 330:550–556.

13. Schneider EL, Guralnik JM. The aging of America: The impact on health care costs. *JAMA.* 1990; 263:2335–2340.

14. Fries JF. Aging, natural death, and the compression of morbidity. *N Engl J Med.* 1980; 303:130–135.

15. Branch L, Jette A, Evashwick C, Polansky M, Rowe G, Diehr P. Toward understanding elders' health service utilization. *J Community Health.* 1981; 7(2):80–92.

16. Gilbert GH, Branch LG, Orav J. An operational definition of the homebound. *Health Serv Res.* 1992; 26:787–800.

17. Weissert WG. Estimating the long-term care population: Prevalence rate and selected characteristics. *Health Care Financing Review.* 1985; 6(4):83–91.

18. Long Term Care Resources. In: Kane RL, Ouslander JG, Abrass IB, eds, *Essentials of Clinical Geriatrics,* 2nd ed. New York, NY: McGraw-Hill; 1989; p. 413.

19. Elston JM, Koch GG, Weissert WG. Regression-adjusted small area estimates of functional dependency in the noninstitutionalized American population age 65 and over. *Am J Public Health.* 1991; 81:335–343.

20. Cornoni-Huntley J, Brock DB, Ostfeld AM, Taylor JO, Wallace RB.

Established Populations for Epidemiologic Studies of the Elderly: A Resource Data Book. Bethesda, Md: National Institute on Aging; 1986. NIH Publication No. 86-2443.

21. Branch LG, Wetle TT, Scherr PA, Cook NR, Evans DA, Hebert LE, Masland EN, Keough ME, Taylor JO. A prospective study of incident comprehensive medical home care use among the elderly. *Am J Public Health.* 1988; 78:255–259.

22. Rice DP, LaPlante MP. Medical expenditures for disability and disabling comorbidity. *Am J Public Health.* 1992; 82:739–741.

23. Manton KG, Corder LS, Stallard E. Estimates of change in chronic disability and institutional incidence and prevalence rates in the U.S. elderly population from the 1982, 1984, and 1989 National Long Term Care Survey. *J Gerontol.* 1993; 48(4):S153–S166.

24. Stone RI, Murtaugh CM. The elderly population with chronic functional disability: Implications for home care eligibility. *Gerontologist.* 1990; 30:491–496.

25. Jackson ME et al. Eligibility for publicly financed home care. *Am J Public Health.* 1992; 82:853–856.

26. Benjamin AE. Determinants of state variations in home health utilization and expenditures under medicare. *Med Care.* 1986; 24:535–547.

27. Welch HG, Wennberg DE, Welch WP. The use of Medicare home health care services. *N Engl J Med.* 1996; 335:324–329.

28. Harris T, Kovar MG, Suzman R, Leinman JC, Feldman JJ. Longitudinal study of physical ability in the oldest-old. *Am J Public Health.* 1989; 79:698–702.

29. Guralnik JM, LaCroix AZ, Branch LG, Kasl SV, Wallace RB. Morbidity and disability in older persons in the years prior to death. *Am J Public Health.* 1991; 81:443–447.

CHAPTER 10

Meeting the Demand for Home Health Care Services in a Complex and Changing World

A s we've seen, the demand created by people needing home care is formidable. Studying provider supply, plus the amount of home care now given, shows us the work lying ahead. First of all, most paid home care is given by home health agencies, not by physicians. Supported by Medicare and Medicaid, home health care has grown enormously in 30 years. Table 10.1 shows the amount of home health agency care recently deployed.

Home health accounted for $15 billion, or 8% of 1995 Medicare payments. Medicare-certified agencies numbered 8,747 by 1995, compared with 1,753 in 1967. In 1994 there were 255,000 registered nurses in home care, with 35,000 licensed practical nurses, 48,000 physical therapists, and 171,000 home health aides. Nursing (47%) and personal care dominate visits. Social workers (<1%), and physical (9%), speech (1%), and occupational therapists(1%) play smaller roles.[1] Registered nurses in home care outnumber all U.S. primary care physicians. And because home care is less than 10% of physician work (house calls being less than 1%) physicians currently play a minor role in the actual delivery of home care.

Home care is also substantial for Medicaid, being 5% of 1993 expenses, compared with hospitals (27%), nursing homes (25%), and physicians (7%). In 1992, when Medicare spent $7.4 billion on home care, 109 mil-

TABLE 10.1 Medicare Home Health Agency Services

Year	Persons served*	Visits*	Visits per person	Visits per 1,000 med. enrollees	Payments $ millions
1974	393	8,070	21	340	141
1980	957	22,428	23	788	662
1986	1,600	38,359	24	1,208	1,795
1992	2,506	132,220	53	3,714	7,397

Source: Health Care Financing Administration, 1993.
*Thousands of persons.

lion Medicaid visits cost $4.8 billion, up from $1.1 billion in 1985, whereas the number of Medicaid home care recipients only doubled. Medicaid pediatric home care is also noteworthy. Most of the $4.8 billion spent in 1992 went to adults, but $177 million was spent on children under age 6, and another $197 million was spent on people aged 6 to 20.[2]

High-tech home care is one of the fastest-growing home care markets. In 1993 infusion therapy (62%), dialysis (29%), and respiratory therapy, including ventilator care (9%), cost $5.8 billion.[3] Durable home medical equipment costs were $14 billion, compared with $16 billion for home health care according to the U.S. Commerce Department. There are billion-dollar discrepancies because data come from many public and private sources. Still, total 1993 home care spending was about $33 billion.[4]

Specific conditions like cancer, emphysema, renal failure, stroke, and orthopedic surgery are among the driving forces behind home care use.[5] But as we saw in chapter 9, home care use increases most dramatically with age and functional limitations. The 1987 National Medical Expenditure Survey (NMES) yielded the data in Table 10.2.

Some functional deficits are overcome by equipment alone, as shown in Table 10.3. The National Long-Term Care Survey found 5 million community-dwelling elders with disability and divided help into categories: human vs. equipment.[6]

The direct fiscal impact on care recipients must always be recognized. In 1982, when $4 billion was spent on home care for 1.2 million people with chronic conditions, nearly $1 billion was out-of-pocket, an average of $164 per month for those users with out-of-pocket costs. The 850,000 persons with five or six ADL impairments paid $439 monthly.[7]

Other factors combine to shape home care delivery. Though home

TABLE 10.2 In-Home Service Visits (All Types)

	Age	Persons	Users	Visits/user
	40–64	60 million	1 million	38
	65–74	16 million	1 million	56
	75–84	8 million	1 million	67
	> 85	2 million	600,000	71
ADL deficits				
	0	227 million	3 million	13
	1	5 million	1 million	43
	2	5 million	1 million	61
	≥ 3	3 million	1 million	102

TABLE 10.3 1989 Elderly Users of Assistance at Home

	Type of functional deficit			
	IADL only	1–2 ADL	3–4 ADL	5–6 ADL
Equipment only	176,653	413,293	39,856	1,405
Personal assistance only	810,997	226,789	38,380	42,141
Equipment and personal assistance	293,886	1,336,859	1,000,828	804,899
Total	**1,360,227**	**1,993,353**	**1,079,064**	**848,435**

health agency care is widely available, access is limited for rural individuals and for urban dwellers in high-crime areas, as discussed later in this chapter. Federal skilled home health benefits are also intermittent, tied to acute illness. Although understandable in view of rising costs, this policy has hindered longitudinal care in complex cases and may promote expensive cycles of acute illness, partial recuperation, discontinuous care, and recurrent acute illness, a concern now being studied. Home health agency growth has been so great and there is so much potential demand that government now seeks to control growth and be more certain of appropriate use.[8]

DETERMING THE NUMBER OF MEDICAL HOME CARE PROVIDERS NEEDED

One "missing link" in home care has been medical providers like physicians and other professional care providers (e.g., nurse practitioners or physician assistants). Several factors will affect the future needs for such medical providers. For example, if functionally impaired people are concentrated in group dwellings, we will need fewer providers. Or if society espouses a lower standard of care for the elderly and functionally impaired, or establishes policies that discourage home care, the demand will be less.

In chapter 9, we noted the critical importance of specifying medical need; we cannot extend the concept of medical care to domains where medical professionals have little power or expertise. Homebound people have diverse needs. Some are clearly medical, like treatment for heart failure. Needs for eyeglasses, dentures, hearing aids, walkers, wheelchairs, and caregivers enfold social dimensions that are less medical. And key issues like income, housing, and transportation affect medical care but are not medical needs. Finally, using new information technology and better targeting may improve home care efficiency and reduce the number of needed medical providers. Still, we will need many more than we now have.

HOW MANY MEDICAL PROVIDERS ARE NEEDED BY THE HOMEBOUND?

In this section I will consider only people who are truly homebound, momentarily setting aside those who are more mobile and yet have home care needs. Let's assume the earlier midrange estimates of homebound persons, defined by functional status and including all ages. In chapter 9 we arrived at a homebound population of 2 million. By 2020 this population may number 3 million and will be proportionately older.

Next, we must estimate the frequency of house calls and the amount of medical care management work. The second wave of the (NMES) provides some help. Of noninstitutionalized elderly persons, 85% lived in densely populated areas (SMSAs). Among those with excellent or good health, 83% had ambulatory physician visits, and of those with some visits, the average number was 8. Of those in fair or poor health, 93% had

TABLE 10.4 Annual Physician Visits by Limitations in Functional Status

Age	None Male	None Female	Limited in minor activities Male	Limited in minor activities Female	Limited in major activities Male	Limited in major activities Female	Cannot perform major activities Male	Cannot perform major activities Female
45–54	3.0	3.9	4.6	8.3	5.9	11.5	12.2	23.1
55–64	3.1	4.2	6.3	8.3	7.6	10.7	10.3	19.5
65–74	3.6	5.2	6.5	6.9	7.4	10.3	8.3	13.4
≥74	5.0	4.9	*	5.7	7.1	6.9	9.3	9.8

Source: National Center for Health Statistics. *J Am Geriatr Soc.* 1984; 32(9):670–675.

* Cell too small for accurate estimate.

some ambulatory visits, averaging 12 per year. These contacts occurred in a fee-for-service system, where patients have modest out-of-pocket expenses, encouraging increased volume.[9] A similar pattern is seen in Table 10.4.

Here the functionally impaired had many annual physician contacts, and the frequency of visits for those with most severe impairment diminished with age. This may simply reflect trouble reaching physicians, but it is also possible that the goals of medical care change for very dependent people as they age. Patients and physicians may recognize the approach of life's end and look less to medicine for resolution. Perhaps the 12 medical contacts reported in the NMES are enough.

It also appears that many functionally impaired people managed to encounter physicians despite a paucity of house calls. If so, is there truly an access problem? Here these data run thin. We do not know if contact was made in emergency rooms, physician offices, or other settings. We do not know how difficult it was to make contact, whether the contact was timely in relation to clinical need, or whether continuity of care was preserved. And those "hidden," socially isolated homebound people, missed by surveys but familiar to home care physicians, are excluded.

The frequency of physician contacts by the least healthy NMES and National Center for Health Statistics (NCHS) subgroups also recall mandatory contacts in nursing homes. A physician or an affiliated professional provider must see each patient no less often than every 2 months, after an initial period with three monthly visits. Likewise, Medicare requires physicians to review home care treatment plans every 60 days, again pushing physicians to actively supervise care of frail, medically ill people. These regulations, right or wrong, represent distilled experience from thousands of providers and millions of patients and suggest a need for continuous medical care.

Social HMOs, which enroll Medicare beneficiaries in a capitated arrangement covering long-term care along with acute and ambulatory care, offer another perspective. Physicians' financial incentives for increased volume are removed, whereas patients' small disincentives (co-payments) are also reduced. According to colleagues, typical Medicare managed care patients have 6 to 8 annual outpatient physician contacts, whereas frail seniors over age 75 average 10 to 12 contacts.

DETERMING PROVIDER HOUSE CALL CAPACITY AND CASELOAD

Some of the most authentic data about capacity may be the experience of home care specialists. The British have a more established home care tradition.[10] British general practitioners make house calls, comprising 5% to 12% of outpatient contacts.[11,12] The denominator for this activity is a patient list of between 1,000 and 3,500 people, with about 30 office visits per weekday. There are 20 to 25 weekly house calls, including nights and weekends, and weekly travel time is about 5 hours.

Then consider the Medical College of Virginia (MCV) Home Care Program experience. When we have room for new patients, we enroll people who are homebound (impossible or very difficult to reach the clinic) if they live within 15 miles of the hospital and accept a program physician as their primary provider. The core team includes 3 physicians, who constitute 1.2 full-time equivalents (FTEs), 2 full-time nurse practitioners, 1 half-time social worker, and 1 secretary/patient advocate. House calls, both scheduled and urgent, are made during weekday daylight hours. After hours, telephone coverage is provided by the faculty group practice, but these covering physicians do not make house calls.

Generally, the patients are old, poor, and frail. Mean age is 74 (range 26–103), 71% are women, 80% are African American, and 40% are poor

TABLE 10.5 Functional Dependency of New MCV Home Care Patients

Function, best day	No.	%
Totally bedridden	112	17
Bed-to-chair with maximal assistance	143	22
Bed-to-chair with minimal assistance	53	8
Bed-to-chair with no assistance	40	6
Ambulatory with assistance (human/equipment)	187	29
Ambulatory without assistance	98	15

enough to qualify for Medicaid. About one-third are also open to home health agency skilled care at any one time, providing extra eyes and ears but also reflecting degree of illness. Patients live in various settings: private homes (60%), adult homes (10%), and senior apartment complexes (30%). Thus, the patients are geographically dispersed, which increases travel time and decreases caseload. The 647 patients listed in the MCV Home Care database since 1987 are characterized by functional dependency on enrollment, demonstrated in Table 10.5.

Hospitalizations are common, recently averaging one admission and 10 inpatient days per program-patient-year. Death is the most common cause for leaving the program. Of those who have left MCV Home Care, 67% have died, half at home and half in the hospital. Few patients have a clearly terminal prognosis at entry, yet the mean duration of enrollment is only 15 months. Approximately 31% of the patients die within their first year, and 41% are dead by 2 years. These people are seriously ill; they require active care coordination and frequent personal attention. Thus, our experience mirrors formal studies showing that ADL deficits often predict mortality better than medical diagnoses.

Efficiency also affects capacity. Several factors promote efficiency at MCV Home Care. One is constant pressure to enroll new patients. Staff experience and familiarity with the patients help determine visit frequency and the urgency of unplanned visits in response to phone calls. The day's visits are also grouped geographically to reduce "windshield time," and we have organized methods for managing information and arranging other services.

In some ways our efficiency is impaired. We lack state-of-the-art cellular phones and computerized information handling, and we spend time compensating for the complexity of a large urban medical center. Furthermore, many patients have extensive social needs that drive care management work and consume provider energy. I believe new technologies could enhance our efficiency, but I estimate that the improvement would be a modest 25%.

Given this background, we can consider the frequency of MCV Home Care house calls and provider time for delivery and coordination of care as measures of capacity for home care providers. Our average patient is seen 10 times a year, ranging from 2 to 33. This average, derived from an admittedly selected population and the practice of one small provider group, matches the parameters suggested by the NMES data and by nursing home and home health regulations. Average miles per visit in our largely urban setting (6) and average visit time (60 minutes, including travel) have been consistent. At a brisk pace, five visits fill a half day as illustrated below.

For those less familiar with home care practice it may be useful to follow a morning's work. I designed my route to end at the hospital, intending to see 7 patients. Leaving my house at 7:15, I made a routine visit to VW, a 25-year-old with cerebral palsy and seizures, who survived a serious bout with pneumonia a few years ago. I planned a 6-month checkup, certification for home services, and drawing blood for a Dilantin level. This required a femoral vein puncture because VW has tiny veins and fights having her blood drawn, not understanding what is being done. Unexpectedly, VW had been sick for 2 days and appeared to have early pneumonia. Her mother preferred treatment at home. Blood was drawn, put in the cooler, and VW's mother was instructed about antibiotics. The visit took 45 minutes.

Next came DT, a new patient. This 46-year-old had Down's syndrome, severe congenital heart disease, moderate kidney failure, newly diagnosed tuberculosis, and severe gout. He had been hospitalized three times in recent months and had just been discharged a week earlier. DT now had nine medicines in two conflicting sets of prefilled medication boxes, and his gout medicines were stopped in the hospital for unknown reasons. He had suffered from discontinuous care. His functional status had declined abruptly. Now he was bedfast, in so much pain from gouty joints that he resisted being turned or bathed. Previously, he got out of bed unassisted, independently used his wheelchair and bedside commode, and charmed the nurses.

DT now had acute gout in both knees, and a grade III pressure ulcer under his left heel, which was missed by both the hospital physicians and the home health nurse. His heart rate was high at 120, and he was unusually drowsy though answering questions appropriately. I drew blood, put it in the cooler, phoned in orders for protective foot coverings and a special mattress, and asked my office to gather information about the prior medical management. I also spent a few minutes counseling DT's caregiver, his remarkable 88-year-old mother. It was nearly 10 a.m. The visit took over 90 minutes. I called in VW's antibiotics now that the pharmacy was open and ordered a home X ray to confirm her pneumonia.

The next two patients were at a nearby adult home. One man needed injections in his knees to relieve chronic arthritic pain, and his blood pressure had to be checked after a medication change. His knees are difficult to puncture, requiring my presence rather than that of the nurse practitioner who usually sees him. This visit took 30 minutes. Down the hall was WM, recently hospitalized for a bladder infection, impaction, and acute arthritis in her knee. Together, these made her bedfast and incontinent, a "dead weight." Now I was glad to see that she was much better, though her blood pressure was very high and I changed her medication. This visit lasted less than 15 minutes. It was 11:15.

With with two acute problems needing resolution (VW and DT), I postponed two stable patients and drove by the office, handing lab specimens to the secretary who met me at the curb. The seventh scheduled patient needed a brief checkup plus a blood test because he was on high-dose potassium replacement for severe diarrhea. His veins are hard to find, and it took two attempts, but I was back at the hospital by 12:30, having seen five patients in 5.5 hours, including one new patient. In this time I worked quickly, used my home care experience, and drove only 16 miles.

Thus, for me, 10 housecalls make a very full day. Rushing, I have made 12 or 13 visits, a pace I cannot easily sustain. More reasonable would be 8 or 9 daily visits, allowing time for paperwork, charting, and answering pages. So house calls themselves take more than twice as long as office encounters, where general internists see over 20 patients per day. Further differentiating home care from office practice is the case management work before and after the house call, work that consumes as much as 35% of one's time (see chapter 2). At 10 house calls per day there is little time for case management unless one does the work while driving and has a budget to support a large cellular phone bill.

Using the above parameters, one urban home care physician—working 250 days a year, making 9 visits per day, averaging 10 visits per patient per year, and spending 35% of the week on care management that does not involve direct patient contact or travel—could handle 150 homebound patients living in separate dwellings.

These assumptions can be partially validated. Virginia primary care physicians reported average house call time at 52 minutes, including travel. This was elicited by the question, "How much time, in minutes, would you estimate you spend on one home visit, including travel time."[13] In a national sample, family physicians and internists reporting an average of 36 homebound patients also claimed 4.7 hours per week, or 7% of total work, for telephone and paperwork management related to home care.[14] Although an artificial manipulation, extrapolating to a practice of 150 home care patients would bring time for "care management" work to 19.6 hours, or 32% of a 60-hour work week. And a formal time-motion study of the Rochester home care team found 40% of time consumed by activities other than patient contact and travel, as described in chapter 2.

There are other data that must be considered. Adelman reported that 56% of primary care physicians spend between 20 and 40 minutes per house call, 29% spending between 41 and 60 minutes.[15] However, travel time and charting were not mentioned in that survey. And Philbrick[16] reported a 48-minute average for rural housecalls: 20 minutes for travel and 28 minutes in the home. To make reasonable estimates of work load, it is critical to know the setting and the types of patient problems encountered. Patients with active, complex medical and social problems takes more time and effort than stable chronic care patients. We clearly need more data about physician home care work.

The work of professional providers was explored in chapter 3. Recall that two MCV Home Care nurse practitioners make 65% of all visits, make about 800 visits each per year, and manage a case load of 50 to 70 patients with physician support. They also handle many of the phone calls and much care management. An experienced home care physician might oversee the work of three nurse practitioners caring for sick homebound patients. Capacity is then limited by the physician's need to know the patients personally. This physician could carry some additional cases without nurse practitioner help.

To complete the spectrum of service capacity, consider George Taler's approach in Maryland, where he relies on visiting nurses for both chronic and acute care while he provides longitudinal physician direction. He allows one-half day per week, with five to seven visits per half day, to provide quarterly house calls for 50 or 60 patients. A nurse case manager does most of the care coordination. In this instance the physician's lesser role in acute situations, the larger role for visiting nurses in the absence of professional providers, and the lack of comparative data about the patients and their use of other services all hinder direct comparisons with MCV Home Care. More research is needed.

TOTALING UP THE PROVIDER PICTURE

Let us now return to the earlier estimate of 2 million homebound persons. If patients average 10 annual house calls, if mobile providers can deliver 9 house calls per day, if 35% of the week is consumed with care management, and if providers work 250 days each year, we would need about 14,000 FTEs for house calls to the chronically homebound, and they would deliver 20 million house calls. This also assumes a metropolitan setting. Travel time would increase the number of providers needed in rural locations.

Variations on this model could include more house calls per day, less time for care management, and longer intervals between house calls, all of which would reduce the number of needed providers. For example, if providers could average 12 house calls per day, spend only 25% of their time on care management, and see patients eight times a year, house calls and home care oversight for 2 million persons would require 7,000 FTEs, delivering 16 million house calls. Further reducing annual house calls to six per patient brings us to 5,000 FTEs making 12 million house calls.

Comparing this potential demand to current services is scary. In 1965 internists made 4.8 house calls per week,[17] and in 1966 pediatricians in upstate New York made 15 house calls per week.[18] In 1976, New Jersey family physicians made six house calls per week.[19] However, the house call's decline is undisputed. In 1980 only 0.6% of physician visits occurred in the patient's home.[20] By 1988, 87% of Virginia's adult primary care physicians offered house calls, but they averaged only two per month, and less than 25% made more than one per week.[21] Seventy-six percent of Minnesota family physicians reported house calls in 1988, but only 10% had made two or more in the previous month, and 84% made 15 or fewer in the previous year.[22] Seventy percent of Utah's adult primary care physicians made house calls in 1985 but only at 2.6 visits per month.[23] Nationally, about half of internists and family physicians reported house calls in 1990, more family physicians (65%) making house calls than did internists (44%).[24] The mean annual number was 9 for the entire sample, with 21 by family physicians who made house calls and 16 by internists who made house calls. Adelman's 1991 national survey found that 63% of family physicians, 47% of internists, and 15% of pediatricians made house calls.[15] The average frequency was 1.6 every 2 weeks, or 38 house-calls in a 48-week year with 4 weeks' vacation.

Thus, using the most optimistic figures, if 65% of family physicians each made 30 house calls per year, this would yield 940,000. If 45% of 76,000 general internists each made 25 house calls per year, they would add up to 855,000. If 15% of 45,000 pediatricians made 20 house calls per year, there would be 135,000 pediatric house calls. The total would be about 2 million house calls.

Confirming the survey data, consider that Medicare receives about 1.5 million bills on house call codes each year. Medicaid house call numbers are far smaller. This count is incomplete. There are no reliable data for private insurance, house calls paid for out-of-pocket, or house calls that are never billed. We also know that federal billing data are incomplete because some physicians do not use house call codes and others eschew billing federal carriers, frustrated by scanty reimbursement or lacking awareness of billing procedures. Still, even if we doubled current billings to 3 million, we would fall far short of the need. These underserved patients may never see physicians, may go to physicians' offices at high personal cost, or may see physicians in emergency rooms and other institutional settings, but they clearly are not being seen at home.

To make this exercise even more distressing, extend the calculations to the projected 3 million homebound persons in the year 2020. Using our baseline assumptions, they would need 30 million house calls and 20,000 FTEs. Accepting the leanest assumptions, probably unrealistic and inadequate, they would still need 18 million housecalls and 8,000 FTEs.

The evident shortage of house calls is one issue, but then we must consider the numbers of available physician providers. One study of physician supply indicated that in the year 2000 between 13,000 and 32,000 primary care physician FTEs would be needed for care of the elderly, rising as high as 47,000 by 2020.[25] Limitations in that report prompted a more recent study. Reuben et al. estimated the number of physicians needed for geriatric care, now and in 2030.[26] They stratified the elderly by age and functional impairment and considered whether or not people were institutionalized. Utilization data, all from the mid-1980s, came from the National Nursing Home Study, the National Health Interview Supplement on Aging, the National Ambulatory Care Study, and Medicare. These were augmented by time-motion data from geriatric HMOs and a national physician survey. Three models were developed, using variations in the economy, population, health policy, and technology.

The researchers found a need for 47,000 geriatric primary care physician FTEs in the year 2000. They projected a need by 2020 for 100,000 to 120,000 *total* physician FTEs dedicated to care of the elderly, with a smaller number of geriatricians, ranging from 2,000 to 9,000. Most care would be given by general internists and family physicians, comprising 60% of all physician work. Geriatricians would have specialized roles in education, research, administration, and care of the very frail. Specialists from other disciplines would give 35% of physician care. The 70,000 generalist FTEs needed for geriatric care would be spread across a much larger number of generalists who carried patients both young and old.

For perspective, consider that practicing general internists and family physicians in 1990 altogether numbered only 124,000. There were about 48,000 family physicians (79% office-based), 23,000 general practitioners (90% office-based), and 76,00 general internists (61% office-based) among 615,000 U.S. physicians. Many were involved principally in the care of younger populations. Only 39% of internists' office visits involved geriatric patients.[27] The fraction would be lower for family physicians. Even if 35% of visits to both disciplines involved geriatric patients, the existing providers in these two largest provider groups, not including osteopaths, would deliver only 43,000 FTEs of geriatric outpatient care, far from the 70,000 FTEs needed 25 years hence. Moreover, these future geriatric physicians will likely focus most of their effort on hospitals, nursing homes, community health centers, physician offices, and settings other than home care.

Thus, there is already a serious shortage of physician involvement in geriatric home care, and the gap will certainly expand unless the provider supply changes in both number and preparation. We will also need providers to fill the current large void in home care for younger populations. And finally, remember the home care needs of people who are not chronically homebound, the more mobile office-based patients whose home care needs are also important, albeit less intensive. A primary care physician may spend 3.5 hours per week on home care oversight,[14] including both complex patients and those less severely impaired. At 1 hour of low-intensity home care per week, this would occupy 1,500 FTEs.

It is true that professional care providers could help fill the breach. This approach has conceptual appeal, both clinically and fiscally. Consider a model like MCV Home Care. Nurse practitioners, the professional providers with whom I have worked most closely, can handle an active case-load of about 50 to 70 frail homebound patients, delivering two-thirds of the house calls. If 2 million homebound people were in the care of such teams, we would need about 28,000 professional FTEs. They would deliver 70% of 20 million house calls while team physicians delivered the other 6 million. We would need only 4,000 physician FTEs rather than 14,000. The main problem with this proposition is that there are only about 35,000 nurse practitioners and 32,000 physician assistants in the entire work force. There are only 1,200 gerontologic nurse practitioners. The supply of professional providers is very limited.

Specialized physicians are another possible resource. The Council on Graduate Medical Education estimates that by the year 2000 there will be a surplus of 165,000 physicians, most of them specialists. There is still an active debate about the mix of primary care physicians and specialists and the definition of primary care,[28] but we seem to be moving from a formula with about 35% primary care toward one with 45% primary care.[29] I have certainly seen a healthy excess in consultations and procedures during my young career, driven by convention, by referral patterns, and perhaps by financial self-interest rather than by clinical need. Home care may be a role to consider when redirecting the energies of some specialists.

SELECTED TROUBLE SPOTS: UNDERSERVED AREAS AND MISSING HELPERS

Important external factors influence estimates of supply, and these require exploration. One is the issue of rural areas and underserved urban communities.

Rural Areas

The service capacity calculations above are for urban and suburban home care. Rural home care is a different story. Rural health itself is a large topic, with a complex agenda that has been well covered elsewhere, but some foundations are needed here.

We must first define the dimensions of the term *rural*. For example, I have made many house calls in areas just outside Richmond that I consider rural. Distances between houses are sizable, and there are no nearby physicians' offices. I have also traveled through rural states like West Virginia, Utah, Texas, Montana, and Arizona. There's a stark contrast between the beautiful, arid mesas of Navajo country in northeast Arizona and populous Phoenix, where home care is a growth market.

Formal studies help one properly understand this problem. Braden and Beauregard[30] define "ruralness" and review data showing that many of America's poor live in rural counties with chronically depressed economies. Of 242 such counties, 224 were in the South. They note 1980–1981 National Health Interview Survey data revealing that fair or poor health is more prevalent among rural residents, especially the elderly, compared with nonrural populations. Rowland and Lyons echo the poverty theme. Over half the poor live in rural areas,[31] and 18% of rural residents are impoverished. Lack of insurance is relevant to rural home care physicians, as is the fact that the rural poor are more limited by chronic disease. In one report, half of West Virginia family physicians were considering relocating, primarily because of financial jeopardy.[32]

Several studies have documented rural physician shortages, especially in the northern Great Plains, northern New England, the upper Great Lakes, and the Southeast. In these areas 300,000 persons lived over 25 miles from a physician. According to the NMES,[33] 7% of people live more than 30 minutes drive from their usual source of medical care.

The regional differences are striking. Using 1977 data, Berk studied medical care in Health Manpower Shortage (HMS) areas, affecting 14% of the U.S. population. Twenty-six percent lived in urban areas, and 27% lived in rural areas. The remainder lived in the periphery of smaller cities or populous nonurban areas. Half of the shortage areas were in the South, where 89% of rural HMS area residents lived, many being members of minority groups. Conversely, 78% of urban HMS area residents lived in the Northeast and the north-central regions.[34] In rural HMS areas, 29% of people traveled over 30 minutes to see physicians. The authors noted that rural residents may have similar problems with access to essentials other than health care, such as food. Thus, distances are an accepted reality when one first chooses a rural life. However, they did not discuss the medical or social implications of later becoming immobilized by unexpected illness in a rural setting.

In 1991 a nonrandom group of rural home health agencies studied by the National Association for Home Care raised similar concerns. One-way travel distances of 60 miles were reported, ranging up to 150 miles. Providers traveled in cars and four-wheel drive vehicles but occasionally used cross-country skis, flat-bottomed boats, airplanes, and horses. Road conditions and staffing were frequent problems. Social work, home aides, and physical, occupational, and speech therapy were especially problematic.

Rural physicians' home care role differs from that of urban colleagues. In Utah, rural and suburban internists, family physicians, and general practitioners make house calls more often than urban physicians do.[23] Rural Virginia physicians also showed a slightly higher propensity to make house calls.[21] Rural Minnesota family physicians were more likely than urban counterparts to make house calls (84% vs. 68%).[22] Adelman's 1991 national primary care physician survey found rural physicians more likely to make house calls.[15] And Keenan[24] found a similar pattern in a 1990 national survey (see Figure 10.1). "Rural" was defined here by counties not in an SMSA.

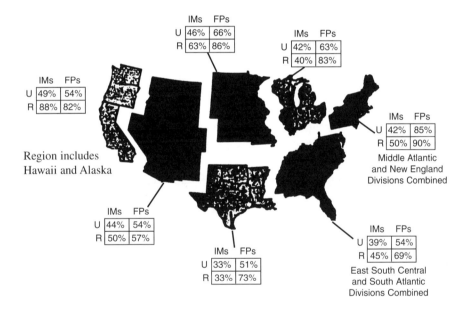

	IMs	FPs
U	46%	66%
R	63%	86%

	IMs	FPs
U	42%	63%
R	40%	83%

	IMs	FPs
U	49%	54%
R	88%	82%

	IMs	FPs
U	42%	85%
R	50%	90%

Middle Atlantic and New England Divisions Combined

Region includes Hawaii and Alaska

	IMs	FPs
U	44%	54%
R	50%	57%

	IMs	FPs
U	33%	51%
R	33%	73%

	IMs	FPs
U	39%	54%
R	45%	69%

East South Central and South Atlantic Divisions Combined

Figure 10.1 Percentage of physicians making home visits, by specialty and census division, IMs indicates internal medicine physicians, FPs, family practice physicians; U, Urban; and R, rural.

TABLE 10.6 Percentage of Physicians Reporting Service Readily Available

Home health service	Nonrural	Rural
Skilled nursing	85	84
Physical/occupational/speech therapy	68	52
Medical social service	68	51
Appliance/equipment	83	73

I found only one detailed report about the clinical aspect of rural house calls. Philbrick described the Orange County Clinic in a Virginia county of 21,000.[16] During 26 months, 138 house calls were made to 47 of 2,539 individuals in the practice. Thus, there were 2.9 visits per patient among those receiving house calls, ranging up to 22 visits. A few children received house calls, but most involved older patients, an average one-way distance of 7 miles, ranging up to 50 miles. Over half the patients were not permanently homebound but were seen at home for acute illness or acute exacerbations of chronic illness. In retrospect, physicians considered 80% of the house calls appropriate. They felt that nurses could have handled 3% and another 3% could have been resolved on the phone. Of the 14% deemed inappropriate, reasons for the visits were usually patient or caregiver convenience.

The 1990 national physician survey also gathered data on referrals to home care agencies in rural areas.[14] Rural physicians ($N = 230$) reported more frequent referrals than did nonrural counterparts ($N = 931$) and were more likely to be home health agency medical directors. However, despite their apparent reliance on home care, rural physicians reported less availability of services (see Table 10.6).

An analysis of 1987 Medicare data confirms this lack. Rural areas showed a slightly lower overall volume of home care services than urban areas, and rural home health agencies less often provided physical or occupational therapy or social work.[35] Episodes of home care were also much longer, with less frequent visits.[36]

Certain issues are critical in rural home care. One is travel. Distances are greater, and this is compounded by the challenge of getting around. Roads may be poorly marked, and people may rely on landmarks like "the big oak tree." There may be no direct route from point A to point B. It's easy to get lost, and extremes of weather can make country roads impassable.

A related feature lacking in many rural areas is the transport system on which physicians in more populous areas rely for office-based care of the functionally impaired. Ambulance and wheelchair van service is less available. Combined with a community-oriented mindset among rural physicians, this may be one of the reasons that rural physicians make more house calls.

Although there may be reasons to make more house calls, the rural physician or professional provider may also be the "only game in town," making it difficult to leave the office unattended. And there is the related problem of covering costs, so activities like house calls that are time-consuming and inadequately reimbursed add to an already serious fiscal handicap.

When rural physicians make house calls, other issues arise. I have walked on hard-packed earthen floors in Richmond and visited homes with ancient wiring, no electricity, or poor plumbing, but this happens rarely. In truly rural settings, lack of basic services may hinder home care practice. This includes telephone service. Having no telephone makes home care much more difficult.

Thus, rural home care is challenging. It is a relief that only 20% of the U.S. population lives in rural areas, depending on how one defines "rural," and as few as 4% live in rural HMS areas. And it is encouraging that the Agency for Health Care Policy and Research has recently funded a $2 million study dedicated to understanding home care for America's 7.6 million rural elderly.

Nonrural Underserved Areas

Compared with people living in more affluent sections of the city, many of my home care patients in central Richmond live in an area of relative physician shortage. Like many cities, Richmond has a physician excess and a local maldistribution. Berk found that 26% of people in HMS areas lived in urban settings. Having witnessed the desolation of inner-city communties firsthand, I understand the plight of the urban underserved. Geography is less problematic, but provider maldistribution remains serious.

Urban home care brings its own unique challenges. Finding apartments can be difficult because many public housing developments are poorly labeled. Parking can be problematic. Once inside, concern for provider safety, discussed earlier, is an issue. The prevalence of narcotics, assumed criminal activity, and fear of violent crime can discourage house calls. Finally, the work environment—noisy, sometimes unclean, and often pest-ridden—may be unappealing. These factors tend to increase the gap between needs and services.

The Hidden Invalid Problem

Among the 8.8 million elderly people living alone, described by the Commonwealth Fund Commission on Elderly People Living Alone, are many who are isolated yet have great difficulty with self-care. Some are found and helped by outreach programs like the Living-at-Home Programs[37] or New York's St. Vincent's Hospital Chelsea Village Program.[38] These are among the most difficult home care patients. They are invisible to community long-term care systems until they are reported by a neighbor, landlord, or family member. Many are demented, alcoholic, or chronically mentally ill. They adhere tenaciously to familiar environments, often long after their position is untenable. Care of one such patient requires several times the work needed by someone with similar medical needs but better supports. It takes a strong community network for case finding and a very dedicated group of providers to serve this population.

The Caregiver Supply Problem

Because unpaid informal caregivers do most of the work in home care, their supply is critical. Stone provides details with a 1982 study.[39] Of 2 million elders needing help with one or more ADLs, 1.8 million received informal caregiving. Caregivers tended to be female (72%), averaging 57 years of age, and 35% were elderly. Spouses were the predominant sole caregivers (55% to 60%), followed by adult daughters. One-third of caregivers were themselves in "fair or poor" health. The median duration of caregiving was 1 to 4 years (44%), 20% reporting 5 years or more. Eighty percent provided unpaid assistance 7 days per week. Average effort was 1–2 hours per day for 57%, 3–4 hours per day for 19%, and 5 or more hours per day for 16%, with a mean of 4 hours. These busy caregivers had competing demands. Thirty-one percent were employed, and one-fifth had child care responsibilities. Some had left the labor force to become caregivers. Twenty percent had reduced work hours, changed schedules, or taken time off work.

Recalling the previous chapter, we know that the number of frail elders is increasing far faster than the number of potential caregivers, a situation further compounded by the number of women entering the work force rather than staying at home where they could be caregivers. Where will this leave home care physicians who rely heavily on information and support from these caregivers, just as the caregivers rely on the physicians for support and advice?

POSSIBLE FUTURE EFFECTS
ON SUPPLY AND DEMAND

Because social support is so vital, one option is to redesign communities, including more group living facilities. Life care communities and senior apartment complexes will become home for more senior citizens. About 15% of those over age 75 in the year 2000 and 25% of this subpopulation in 2020 could afford life care settings as presently financed (see chapter 8 ref. 11). Whether they will choose them remains to be seen. For less affluent elders, the "high risers," or senior apartment buildings, are often a haven in a dangerous and difficult world. Concentrating the frail elders will create opportunities for efficient care,[40] but it will also disrupt some patient-physician relationships and lessen continuity.

Another force that will shape the future of home health care is consumer preference. Patients and their overextended caregivers will press for more services at home. The reduced productivity of caregivers who lose time from work may drive more formal home care. Most of the patients are chronically impaired, so the economic impact will be ongoing and substantial. As these demands create political pressure and market forces, physician home care should follow. Ultimately, I believe home care will be seen as a less expensive alternative for delivering medical care, once transportation costs, the delays caused by such patients in the physician's office, and the other hidden costs of the current system are fully exposed. And as providers assume more financial risk, home care will have an ever higher priority.

THE "FRAYED EDGE": MORAL AND ETHICAL
CONSIDERATIONS IN A TIME OF SHORTAGE

The importance of social supports is never so apparent as when they are inadequate, which leads to a variety of moral and ethical problems in home care. This has great relevance to the foregoing discussion of matching services and needs because of the amount of work these cases require. Callahan suggests that the goals of medicine have become too broad, going beyond reasonable efforts to promote physical or psychological health and trying to encompass "happiness." He suggests that medicine must better define its limits in relation to the social context in which medical practice exists.[41] He indicates that we have collectively come to expect too much of biomedical interventions in old age and that we want to receive more than we can collectively afford. In home care the tension between the physician's medical role and the broader social context becomes evident when patients continue to live at home after their needs exceed the available help. Frequently, the home care physician faces ethical dilemmas and may be asked to use medical authority in resolving primarily social conflicts. The home care physician then operates in the ill-defined interface between medicine and society. This is the "frayed edge." It is difficult terrain.

Following are MCV Home Care cases that illustrate the kinds of problems these physicians encounter. The work of overseeing routine home health agency care or chronic care house calls, the work of terminal care, or even of directing high-tech medical care may all pale when compared with the work in a case with dominant social elements.

One common debate centers on patient safety. SB was blind but slowly ambulatory, his urinary catheter bag in hand. His blind wife, JB, was completely bedfast from paraplegia plus massive obesity, which made care difficult. She was rolled from side to side to clean her chronically inflamed skin, and she lived permanently in their bed. Both did well on mental status tests, but their judgment was dubious. There had been two fires in the home, and they were saved only by luck. Nursing home placement was advised, and home health nurses repeatedly asked me to intervene, but SB and his wife refused to leave. I spent much time discussing with my home care colleagues the medico-legal issues related to overriding people's rights.

Another debate involves the high cost of medically rescuing such people. After JB died, the elderly diabetic SB, with his many medical problems, lived alone. He was helped in the mornings by a Medicaid personal care aide who spent most of her time watching TV. A cousin allegedly stayed with him at night but was inconstant. SB was an obstinate, demanding person, who spent most of his day in a chair and would not restrict his diet despite uncontrolled diabetes. Eating was his chief pleasure, and home glucose monitoring was impossible for this blind man who had alienated his family, so little could be done for the diabetes. SB also had a chronic internal bladder catheter because of prostate obstruction for which he, fearful of complications, had refused surgery. The catheter caused frequent bouts of severe pain, many phone calls to MCV Home Care, many house calls, dozens of emergency room visits for catheter changes, and hundreds of urgent home nursing visits. Eventually, SB's cancerous prostate forced the definitive treatment we had advised, and the pain stopped. Months later he died at home, found one morning in his favorite chair with a piece of cheese in hand. Other similarly ill MCV Home Care patients, living in far less comfortable surroundings, have received excellent care from their families. These contrasts are compelling.

The next problematic medical-social issue I would mention is socially unacceptable behavior by demented patients. After her husband died, AD lived alone in an old building used for low-rent apartments. A neighborhood friend checked on her and did her shopping, being her principal link to the world. The memorabilia of a lifetime surrounded and anchored her. AD was immobilized by heart failure, arthritis, and weak leg veins that caused foot swelling and skin ulcers at her ankles. She was unable to reach her feet to apply dressings. Though sociable, AD had dementia that was slowly worsening. Only occasionally would she take the few medicines we recommended, and she would never elevate her legs to reduce the swelling. Our medical interventions were relatively ineffectual, and our role was to watch over her.

The apartment was appalling. Urine permeated every surface. The kitchen was drab. A small greasy frying pan held day-old food. Yesterday's Meals-on-Wheels container sat on the table. Roaches roamed uninhibited. The bedroom was mostly filled by the bed, the sheets filthy, the covers piled with her belongings. Adjacent was the bathroom, its floor covered with dried feces and toilet paper from times when AD had been too slow to reach the commode. The odor permeated into the external hallway. Still, AD refused to leave. We debated forcing her to leave by court order, but we had to admit that she seemed happy and that there was no imminent danger. Adult Protective Services concurred. She was seen by our team 67 times during 4 years of home care.

AD's landlord saw things differently. Though he wanted the rent money she paid, he often threatened eviction, so we stayed ready for the day when the police would knock at her door, creating an emergency. Physically and mentally, AD was completely helpless. By default, MCV Home Care had become AD's final advocate, and with a few days' notice we found her a new place to stay when she was ultimately evicted.

The case of FH raises the questions of how to define a minimum quality standard for family care and of who should draw that line. This 83-
year-old woman suffered the third of several strokes. Previously, she cared
for herself. Now she was unresponsive and bedbound, fed through a
gastrostomy, and maintained with an indwelling urinary catheter. She had
a large sacral bedsore, acquired in the hospital. The primary caregiver was
a granddaughter, who worked evenings in a nursing home, helped by a
daughter who was raising her own family nearby. Despite three nursing
visits per week, the wound was worsening. The care was barely adequate
by some observers' standards and unacceptable to others. A hospital inpatient team was horrified by FH's condition when she was admitted for an
infection. Without consulting MCV Home Care, they forcefully told the
family that FH should be in a nursing home.

When we asked the family members why they wanted the responsibility of home care, they gave these reasons. First was loyalty. FH had cared
for her children and grandchildren when they were helpless; now they felt
obliged to care for her. Next was an administrative problem with Medicaid
coverage for nursing home care, related to old insurance policies that were
lost in the attic. Also, the granddaughter noted that many nursing homes
where she had worked did not give patients like FH very good care.
Finally, there was peer pressure: "People will talk if we put her in a home.
They don't offer to help after they say we should keep her at home, but
they would talk if we put her away."

At home, FH was not turned or bathed often enough, and she missed
some feedings. In a nursing home, some aspects of care would improve,
but the outcome would inevitably be poor. She had lost too much neurological function with the strokes, and her diabetic skin would never heal.
Other complications would follow. FH did not appear to be suffering. Then
the care started to improve, and the family members resolved some of their
internal discord. The decision to keep FH at home seemed reasonable, and
our time was probably well spent.

With FH we were concerned about unintentional neglect, but one also
encounters cases of possible abuse. A lawyer colleague on the board of
the Area Agency on Aging asked me for medical consultation in the case
of BN. The lawyer was BN's pro bono court-appointed guardian, and she
was an empathic, fair-minded person whose opinion I respected. BN was
a chronic alcoholic woman who became demented to the point where
neighbors did her shopping and brought the alcohol and cigarettes she
craved. Boarders rented rooms in BN's house. Many were transients; people stole her money and mistreated her. Still, BN claimed she was happy

and wanted to stay at home, in part because moving meant she could no longer drink. The guardian considered the situation untenable and wanted medical help with forced placement if no treatable conditions were found.

Because BN refused to leave home for evaluation, I met the lawyer at BN's Oregon Hill house one early fall evening. BN admitted us, seeming slightly suspicious of our purpose. I asked if we could sit in the kitchen. On the way she paused to lift her dress and urinate on the linoleum floor. She proved moderately demented, incapable of reliably making informed decisions, and she became irritable when we suggested that she consider moving.

After my evaluation, I asked the guardian about the degree of urgency. She made a strong case for chronic abuse and neglect despite steadfast efforts to intervene, so we called a judge, and I requested hospital commitment for psychiatric evaluation, knowing that institutional placement would follow and BN would leave Oregon Hill for the last time later that evening. As I headed home and when I visited BN in the hospital the next morning, I felt pangs of guilt and some sadness. I later learned that BN had quickly adapted to new surroundings in an adult home, perhaps sheltered from her loss by her poor memory. This made me feel less traitorous.

PREPARING TO FACE ETHICAL ISSUES IN HOME CARE

When considering the tension between medical home care and its societal context, *Ethical Conflicts in the Management of Home Care: The Case Manager's Dilemma*[42] is a helpful resource to which I will refer several times. Following is a discussion of the ethical dimensions seen in cases like those just described. A home care physician must understand these concepts well.

Self-Determination and Decision-Making Capacity

One major issue is balancing the individual's right of self-determination or autonomy against the principle of beneficence or paternalism when deciding whether a person can or should remain at home.[42, chap 4] Is the patient able to make an informed decision about a particular matter? Impaired patients' cognition falls along a spectrum of incapacity.

Incapacity for a complex medical choice involving probabilities and multiple possible outcomes can coexist with capacity for making simpler choices. Specific questions help define capacity, along with objective tests of memory and other cognitive functions. Could the person use the phone to get help? What would happen if a fire started? Can the patient articulate a plan for getting medications, food, and other essentials? A related question is, how much weight should one give to the opinion of a patient with partial impairment? Unlike children who are incapacitated from birth, newly incapacitated adults have a value history that should be considered and that often can be elicited despite dementia or other cognitive impairment.

Further, who determines incapacity? When decisional capacity is impaired, who decides how much patient risk is acceptable? How much of the day, if any, can a dependent adult be left alone? For small families this can be a major problem; caregivers may need to go out, and they sometimes leave vulnerable people unattended. Nurses and social workers are sometimes left to make these decisions without sufficient medical input. Susan Wolf notes instances where precipitous physician judgments of incapacity should also be questioned. Still, I believe that a physician experienced with this process, not always a psychiatrist, should play a central role and that the best decisions come from interdisciplinary teams who have longitudinal relationships with their patients. Once the question of surrogate decision making is raised in court, lines of authority are clear. However, most cases should not involve courts, and wherever they are made, the decisions should be fair.

Caregiver burden and guilt must also be addressed. One must think not only of the current situation but of the alternatives: In what ways would the patient be better served? One must consider the overall prognosis and be biased in favor of care at home. Ideally, everyone with a stake in the situation should participate in a group decision.

This balance of autonomy and beneficence is the most common source of ethical debate in home care and usually involves patients with dementia or other psychiatric impairment of decision making. The dilemma is usually complicated because the degree of impaired capacity and the magnitude of risk are in the "gray zone."

Fiduciary Responsibility

The fiduciary responsibility of care managers is another key topic.[42, chap 5] The perspective of case managers, usually working for public agencies, sometimes differs from that of physicians, recalling our discussion of clinical and financial care management models (see chapter 7). Clinicians have primary fiduciary responsibilities only to their patients, whereas other case managers are responsible to the system for which they work, separate from their responsibility to patients. This is an ethical no-man's-land. As a physician I have experienced this tension. I advocate forcefully for my patients, but I also have important relationships with caregivers, home care professionals, and the guardians of public resources. Suppose my patient wants to remain at home but the price would be severe strain on his ailing wife. Should I pressure her? After years of home care experience, my exclusive fiduciary role to the patient is less easily defined. I am ever more comfortable with this duality as I gain a firmer grasp on relevant ethical and legal principles.

Determining Malign Neglect

One must distinguish abuse or neglect from suboptimal care.[42, chap 7] At what point does sharing an older person's Social Security check to cover a family's household expenses change from a socially just distribution of resources to taking unfair advantage? Is grandma being "chained to the bed" and given substandard care while her money sustains teenagers' recreation or so that her children can keep the house, which would be forfeit if nursing home placement were requested? Or is the family simply making the best of a difficult situation? One must remember that only sometimes would the patient would be better served by institutional care.

Social Pressures

Home care physicians from time to time have to deal with "hermits" or "eccentrics," which leads to considerations of how communities define acceptable human behavior.[42, chap 6] "Hermits" are people who are often competent yet choose lifestyles far off the beaten path. In chapter 2, I mentioned that home care physicians must set aside personal cultural biases before entering patients' homes. Community standards are often the basis for such physician biases. We must remember that supporting eccentrics can enrich a community and define its humanity. As noted in Kane and Caplan, there is a strong literary and cultural history that validates this principle.

Working in a System

I have emphasized that a physician's principal loyalties are to the patient and caregiver, with a secondary responsibility to be a prudent manager of public or common resources. This recalls the question of fiduciary relationships and leads to another ethical dilemma: when to bend or break "the rules." An ethical home care professional, experienced as a manager of personal care services, tells me that clients are sometimes advised to emphasize urinary incontinence even when this is a minor or even nonexistent problem. Then the clients can qualify for paid help which they need and which may even keep them out of nursing homes. Sometimes there is a conflict between official policy and the best course of action,[42, chap 10] and the principle of civil disobedience can support bending or even breaking the rules. Justifiable civil disobedience, however, is accompanied by an obligation to work toward improving the rules.

Justice

The last ethical principle I will retrieve from Kane and Caplan[42, chap 13] is that of "justice." This issue involves fair allocation of resources that are shared and that are limited relative to the need. For example, MCV Home Care sets a limit of 15 miles one-way travel because we can't justify driving past needful patients to serve remote patients with similar needs. Steven Miles offers three rules, paraphrased below, to guide case managers in this moral gray zone: (1) emergent needs must take precedence, (2) fairness to clients' needs preempts fairness to providers, and (3) fairness sometimes requires interpretation of the intent rather than the letter of policies. Miles notes that the world is not fair and will never be fair.

In considering justice, I think too about "aging in place." People choose a place to live and then work hard for many years to create a home. Should these people be moved to places where their needs can be more easily met? Whether the setting is a beach condominium in Florida or the Stonestown or Western Park district of San Francisco, one finds that "people don't want to move again. They want this to be their home until they die."[37] Forcing someone to leave home on medical grounds may also financially burden physicians and hospitals. Patients must have a place to go, so some enter hospitals as "social" admissions for which there is no payment. A nursing home might be more appropriate, but obtaining third-party coverage, screening for need, and finding a space can take weeks or months.

THE IMPACT OF MORAL, ETHICAL, AND SOCIAL CONCERNS ON HOME CARE PHYSICIANS

Social cases wear you down. One such case can consume as much energy as several ordinary home care patients. They are particularly draining for empathic physicians and those with a sense of moral obligation to society. The situations may drag on for months or years in a state of chronic irresolution and precarious instability. There is steady demand for more resources than exist. A major threshold is crossed when permanently leaving home for an institution, imbued with a sense of loss, as well as of foreboding, because nursing homes have a reputation as houses of horror. Physicians must be careful when deciding that institutional care is best, as shown in early studies wherein only 35% of patients referred for placement ultimately required nursing home care. Yet it has been shown that some patients are actually happier in an institution.[43] And physicians can often do little other than to stand ready for the crisis that finally forces closure.

Patients and families pressure physicians to find or authorize additional home care, even though the patients may have exceeded societally defined limits. Some family members urge physicians to intervene against the wishes of patients or other family caregivers. Families become sharply divided. Alternatively, pressure on physicians comes from other professionals who feel that a given situation is untenable. Or physicians themselves may feel a need to intercede yet have their hands tied by patients' resistance. Usually, physicians are working in a gray zone where the patient's capacity for decision making or the patient's degree of endangerment are not clear-cut. This amplifies the stress. A fine judgment is required, and much time passes before one can evaluate the correctness of that judgment.

In general, patients who have cultivated and maintained strong relationships with families and neighbors are well served when frailty comes. People who have alienated those around them or who never formed social bonds pose the greatest problems. They are often inherently difficult, less likable individuals, tempting physicians to disengage. Who should be responsible? Some physicians might feel that people make their own beds in which they must then lie. And forcing people out of their homes against their will requires overriding constitutional rights, which is stressful. On the other hand, if one drops such a case, someone else will inevitably have to pick it up, often at a greater aggregate cost to society. Thus, one may be inclined to persist, to endure, and to wait for resolution.

Sympathy for the patients lessens this strain. I can't count the times I have marveled at the understanding of personal history gained in a short house call. This broader view helps me resist frustration and lessens anxiety created by urgent phone calls asking me to override a patient's autonomy while seeking to serve the patient's best interest or that of society.

REFERENCES

1. Home health agency benefits. *Health Care Financing Review.* 1992 Suppl:137.
2. Statistical report on medical care: Eligibles, payments, and services. Baltimore, Md: Health Care Financing Administration, Bureau of Data Management and Strategy, Office of Program Systems, Division of Medicaid Statistics; 1993. HCFA-2082.
3. Stern EM, Tidd GS. Health care reform's effect on home care: Strategies for survival. *Medical Interface.* May 1994; 85–90.
4. Vladeck BC, Miller NA, Clauser SB. The changing face of long-term care. *Health Care Financing Review.* 1993; 14(4):5–23.
5. Gornick M, Hall MJ. Trends in Medicare use of post-hospital care. *Health Care Financing Review.* 1988; (Suppl): 27–38.
6. Manton KG, Corder L, Stallard E. Changes in the use of personal assistance and special equipment from 1982 to 1989: Results from the 1982 and 1989 NLTCS. *Gerontologist.* 1993; 33(2):168–176.
7. Liu K, Manton KG, Liu BM. Home care expenses for the disabled elderly. *Health Care Financing Review.* 1985; 7(2):51–58.
8. Vladeck BC. Medicare home health initiative. *JAMA.* 1994; 271:1566.
9. Cunningham P, Cornelius L. Use of health care: Findings from the SAIAN and the household survey. Rockville, MD: Agency for Health Care Policy and Research; Public Health Service; (AHCPR Pub. No. 93-0041) 1993.
10. Thomas K, Birch S, Milner P, Nicholl J, Westlake L, Williams B. Estimates of general practitioner workload: A review. *J Royal College Gen Pract.* 1989; 39:509–513.
11. Hallam L, Metcalfe DHH. Seasonal variations in the process of care in urban general practice. *J Epidemiol Community Health.* 1985; 39:90–93.
12. Bucquet D, Jarman B, White P. Factors associated with home visiting in an inner London general practice. *Br Med J.* 1985; 290:1480–1483.
13. Boling PA, Retchin SM, Ellis J, Pancoast SA. Factors associated with the frequency of house calls by primary care physicians. *J Gen Intern Med.* 1991; 6:335–340.
14. Boling PA, Keenan JM, Schwartzberg J, Retchin SM, Olson L, Schneiderman M. Reported home health agency referrals by internists and family physi-

cians. *J Am Geriatr Soc.* 1992; 40:1241–1249.

15. Adelman AM, Fredman L, Knight AL. House call practices: A comparison by specialty. *J Fam Pract.* 1994; 39(1):39–44.

16. Philbrick JT, Connelly JE, Corbett EC. Home visits in a rural office practice: Clinical spectrum and effect on utilization of health care services. *J Gen Intern Med.* 1992; 7:522–527.

17. Altman I, Kroeger HH, Clark DA, Johnson AC, Sheps CG. Office practice of internists. 2: Patient load. *JAMA.* 1965; 193:667–672.

18. Hessel SJ, Haggerty RJ. General pediatrics: A study of practice in the mid-1960's. *J Pediatr.* 1968; 73(2):271–279.

19. Warburton SW, Sadler GR, Eikenberry EF. House call patterns of New Jersey family physicians. *J Fam Pract.* 1977; 4:933–938.

20. *National Health Interview Survey—Physician Visits: Volume and Interval since Last Visit.* Washington, DC: National Center for Health Statistics, 1980; p. 24.

21. Boling PA, Retchin SM, Ellis J, Pancoast SA. The influence of physician specialty on housecalls. *Arch Intern Med.* 1990; 150:2333–2337.

22. Keenan JM, Bland CJ, Webster L, Myers S. The house call practice and attitudes of Minnesota family physicians. *J Am Geriatr Soc.* 1991; 39:1100–1104.

23. Schueler MS, Harris DL, Goodenough GK, Collette L. House calls in Utah. *West J Med.* 1987; 147(1):92–94.

24. Keenan JM, Boling PA, Schwartzberg JG, Olson L, Schneidermann M, McCaffrey DJ, Ripsin CM. A national survey of the home visiting practice and attitudes of family physicians and internists. *Arch Intern Med.* 1992; 152:2025–2032.

25. US Department of Health and Human Services, National Institute on Aging. *Personnel for Health Needs of the Elderly through Year 2020.* Bethesda, MD: Author; 1987. Report to Congress.

26. Reuben DB, Zwanziger J, Bradley TB, Fink A, Hirsch SH, Williams AP, Solomon DH, Beck JC. How many physicians will be needed to provide medical care for older persons? Physicians manpower needs for the twenty-first century. *J Am Geriatr Soc.* 1993; 41:444–453.

27. Woodwell DA. *Advance Data.* Washington, DC: National Center for Health Statistics, Public Health Service, U.S. Department of Health and Human Services; 1992. No. 209.

28. Cooper RA. Seeking a balanced physician workforce for the 21st Century. *JAMA.* 1994; 272:680–687.

29. Weiner JP. Forecasting the effects of health reform on US physician workforce requirement: Evidence from HMO staffing patterns. *JAMA.* 1994; 272:222–230.

30. Braden J, Beauregard K. Health status and access to care of rural and urban populations. National Medical Expenditure Survey Research Findings 18 (AHCPR Pub. No. 94-0031). Rockville, MD: Agency For Health Care Policy

and Research. Public Health Service; 1994.

31. Rowland D, Lyons B. Triple jeopardy: Rural, poor, and uninsured. *Health Serv Res.* 1989; 23:975–1004.

32. Sebert SL. Family physicians' perceptions of health manpower needs in West Virginia. *West VA Med.* 1991; 87:506–509.

33. Beauregard K, Cunningham P, Cornelius L. Access to health care: Findings from the survey of American Indians and Alaska Natives. National Medical Expenditure Survey Research Findings 9 (AHCPR Pub. No. 91-0028). Rockville, Md: Public Health Service, Agency for Health Care Policy and Research.

34. Berk M, Bernstein AB, Taylor AK. The use and availability of medical care in health manpower shortage areas. *Inquiry.* 1983; 20:369–380.

35. Kenney GM. Is access to home health care a problem in rural areas? *Am J Public Health.* 1993; 83:412–414.

36. Kenney GM. Rural and urban differentials in Medicare home health use. *Health Care Financing Review.* 1993; 14(4):39–57.

37. Bogdonoff MD, Hughes SL, Weissert WG, Paulsen E. The Living-at Home program: Innovations in service access and case management. New York, NY: Springer Publishing Co; 1991.

38. Brickner PW, Duque T, Kaufman A, Sarg M, Jahre JA, Maturlo S, Janeski JF. The homebound aged: A medically unreached group. *Ann Intern Med.* 1975; 82(1):1–6.

39. Stone R, Cafferata GL, Sangl J. Caregivers of the frail elderly: A national profile. *Gerontologist.* 1987; 27:616–626.

40. Smith G, Falkenstein J, Engblom P. Community-based geriatric care: Ten years and holding. *J Am Geriatr Soc.* 1994; 42(11): SA66, Abstract.

41. Callahan D. Health care for the elderly: How much is enough? In: *Setting Limits: Medical Goals in an Aging Society.* New York, NY: Simon and Schuster; 1987; pp. 16–17.

42. Kane RA, Caplan AL, eds. Ethical conflicts in the management of home care: The case manager's dilemma. New York, NY: Springer Publishing Co; 1993.

43. Pearlman RA, Uhlmann R F. Quality of life in the elderly: Comparisons between nursing home and community residents. *J Appl Gerontol.* 1988; 7:316–330.

CHAPTER 11

Education for Home Health Care

The preceding chapters have treated the serious shortage of physician home care. If my case is valid, physician education must change, a view supported by policymakers.[1,2,3,4] Education, both of the general public and of health professionals, will prove the foundation on which better care for the functionally impaired and the homebound must be built.

My case is unfortunately typical in many respects. Though I am now a home care expert and advocate, this occurred by accident, the result of a chance meeting and a job opportunity. Despite a humanistic upbringing and strong psychosocial teaching at an excellent medical school, I had no formal education about home care. Residency likewise provided only very limited exposure to home care, without any specific faculty guidance. Furthermore, my experience with frail elders was often confined to treating demented patients who fought as I struggled to insert intravenous needles late at night or whose bedsores I hurriedly debrided during frenetic days. This sort of experience can diminish one's enthusiasm if it is the only geriatrics training one receives, and deep-seated antigeriatric attitudes are still far too prevalent.[5-7]

NEGLECT OF HOME CARE EDUCATION

Along with geriatrics, home care has generally been neglected in physician education, as shown by Robbins,[8] a 1990 national survey by the

Liaison Committee on Medical Education,[9] and recent surveys by Steel[10] and Boling.[11] Despite two decades of recommendations to expand home care education, there has been little progress. Contrasted with their limited preparation for home care, graduates are experienced with acute care and increasingly well prepared for office practice. Even nursing home education is moving forward, while home care lags sadly behind. There are exceptions to this rule, including several experimental or elective experiences plus required activities at a few academic centers.

For example, at the State University of New York, Stony Brook, most students taking a required third-year geriatric module reported wanting to learn more geriatrics, though only 20% felt it should be required.[12] Educators at Mount Sinai reported an increase from 22% to 44% in students who felt that geriatrics should be required after their geriatrics experience.[13] At Duke University the "Aging Game" exposes students to a simulation of disabling conditions. The game has been criticized for emphasizing negative aspects of aging and frightening students, but it has also been effective.[14] And finally, all Boston University fourth-year students must spend a month making house calls with the Home Medical Service,[15] and they give the program positive ratings.

However, even these pioneering programs graduate only a few providers who are truly comfortable with home care and who later practice home care actively. Nor does home care interest and skill necessarily follow investment in geriatric education. Community training programs teach more home care than academic centers do, but the commitment remains modest.[11] And family practice has made home care more integral, compared with training in internal medicine, pediatrics, obstetrics-gynecology, surgery, and psychiatry, whose graduates often direct home care treatment. Yet even in family practice programs the actual home care experience varies widely.

Reasons for neglecting home care are many. More easily justified are considerations of prevalence. Patients use more office care and hospital care than home care, and in general, acuity of illness causes mistakes made in the hospital to have greater immediate consequences than mistakes made in home care. Another factor is the rapid advance of curative technical biomedical services, arguably more appropriate for persons whose prognosis is favorable. Thus, competing curricular priorities make home care a difficult sell. As care moves into the community and the technical capability of home care expands, these arguments are becoming quickly outdated.

Unfortunately, these reasons are not always the chief causes for home care's undernourished educational condition. Lack of glamour, or "sex appeal," is one. Medicine abounds with technological miracles. Tiny platinum wires are placed angiographically into an inoperable aneurysm in a young man's brainstem, removing a lethal threat. Human lymphoid cells are extracted, "taught" to attack tumor cells, and reintroduced, causing advanced cancers to melt. How will home care compete with such riveting successes? Home care also shares the handicaps of generalist fields and nursing homes. Much of the work is seen as routine, and less challenging than problems tackled by subspecialists. Like nursing home work, home care is replete with dementia, incontinence, bedsores, pain, indignity, and death. It is messy.

Students may have other reasons for avoiding the debilitated. Like Scrooge, confronted by Dickens's horrific Ghost of Christmas Yet to Come, young medical learners may subconsciously avoid long-term care, perhaps projecting and then rejecting an abhorrent future that may await them. In long-term care the doctor must also leave a familiar setting and travel. It is inconvenient. Substantial paperwork and bureaucracy are unavoidable. Personal safety may be an issue, and getting lost during house calls has limited educational value. How does one make this appealing?

Not least among the barriers is the question of funding. Unlike other clinical areas, payments for house calls offer no chance of cross-subsidizing education with clinical income. House call teaching necessarily involves a few learners at one time, and patient encounters are lengthy. The impact is high, but the process is inefficient, and home care teaching must always be subsidized. Thus, home care education is endangered when budgets get tight.

Finally and perhaps most important, we lack role models and faculty to teach home care. Without committed faculty, home care has little chance in medical education. Faculty development must therefore be one of the first priorities.

CREATING AND USING OPPORTUNITIES FOR HOME CARE EDUCATION

One hopes that enrolling students open to home care teaching will be a by-product of the current movement toward a larger primary care work force. This will help overcome refractory antigeriatric attitudes. New students will also be increasingly familiar with home care as it is being provided to their aging families. Then, we can make home care learning more appealing. One priority is to nourish altruism. We must start early, when students are receptive. In part the enthusiasm of preclinical students for home care stems from a generic thirst for contact with patients and clinicians. The chance to leave dry classrooms and to experience the different cultures and sometimes eye-opening environments found on house calls is also welcome. In the home one finds people who need you, who are often grateful for your help, and who can teach volumes about the resilience of the human spirit.

Later, interest in home care tends to lie with those entering primary care fields, a self-selected group. Yet other, less motivated students must still learn about home care, and they require different hooks. In an obvious oversimplification one recent survey respondent wrote: "The primary cares love it, the surgeons hate it." To unfairly spotlight one discipline, future orthopedists clearly need home care experience, yet home care is usually not a priority for most of these students. Postsurgical patients' discharge plans would improve if residents were more aware of patient and caregiver needs and more familiar with home care. The same may be true of some full-fledged orthopedists. Learner-centered educational strategies are needed. For example, watching a home care nurse give wound care to a diabetic stroke patient might not interest a surgical resident. However, visiting postsurgical patients to see what physical and occupational therapists can (or cannot) accomplish, learning to use home intravenous antibiotics for osteomyelitis, and seeing caregiver burden firsthand may be interesting to future orthopedists. Following the new critical pathways for joint replacements that rely heavily on home care may be an avenue to pursue.

Many other disciplines should teach home care based on the future professional roles of their graduates. Obstetricians order home terbutaline infusion to stop premature labor. Neonatologists order home bilirubin light therapy with "bili blankets," avoiding prolonged hospital care at the start of life. Pediatricians supervise home ventilator care for premature children. In adult homes and single room occupancy buildings, psychiatrists treat people who used to inhabit chronic mental hospitals. They all need the requisite knowledge and skills.

Home health agencies may become powerful allies in physician education because they need and value informed physician support. Unfortunately, besides lacking basic knowledge of home care, U.S. physicians are currently not very adept at interacting with home care teams. Studies show large discrepancies between physicians' self-reported capability[16] and the perceptions of home health agency colleagues.[17] Young physicians lack supervised experience in working with teams that are remote from the physician's usual workplace. This is ironic because physicians work regularly with interdisciplinary teams in other settings. This situation can change if medical educators form teaching partnerships with other home care professionals.

Finally, home care education is helped by strong leadership. For example, William Hazzard, a prominent geriatrician with much personal magnetism, chairs the Department of Medicine at Bowman Gray. He created a program in which students and residents have required geriatrics experiences, now including home care. The same is true at Boston University. Institutions will not make geriatrics a high priority without strong internal advocacy, and the same is doubly true for home care. And while geriatricians make strong allies for home care educators, linking home care education too tightly with geriatrics is unwise. Geriatricians cannot effectively teach about home respiratory care for children with bronchopulmonary dysplasia. Likewise, home care for premature labor and for young patients with severe psychiatric illness are not geriatric subjects. Leadership and advocacy are critical elements for home care.

WHAT SHOULD BE THE GOALS OF HOME HEALTH CARE EDUCATION?

Before looking at specific home care teaching programs, it is well to define educational goals. The Council on Scientific Affairs of the American Medical Association defined 10 principles to guide home care education.[3] Physicians should:

1. acquire appropriate skills in home health care patient assessment.
2. be able to assess the adequacy of family caregivers and informal care resources.
3. be able to evaluate the efficacy of home health care efforts and contribute to improved quality assurance in home health care.
4. be able to apply home health care principles and guidelines appropriately.
5. Know community resources.
6. Be knowledgeable about cost reimbursement policies in home health care.
7. be knowledgeable about home health care technology.

8. be able to integrate home, office, and hospital care for patients.
9. play an active and major role on the home health care team.
10. demonstrate that they value home health care as a part of their practice.

To these, I would add specific clinical knowledge and skills (see chapter 2). Some home care curricula have been developed. This work is ongoing and starting to accelerate.

CURRENT UNDERGRADUATE (MEDICAL STUDENT) HOME CARE EDUCATION

I will illustrate medical student home care education with details from published descriptions, dividing the accounts for simplicity into undergraduate and postgraduate categories. Admittedly, this lumps preclinical students, who have one set of learning needs, together with clinical students, who are ready to learn about clinical practice. I will also cluster interns, residents, and fellows despite differences in learning objectives at each stage.

Boston University,[18] SUNY at Stony Brook,[12] Albert Einstein,[19] and Harvard[20] have used home care as a venue for teaching students. Very few programs are intensive or mandatory (e.g., Boston University's Home Medical Service), but other medical schools have made serious efforts. At Maryland, 18 students were evaluated after 167 house calls.[21] House calls were part of a 2-month, required fourth-year rotation at the University of California, San Francisco.[22] And though we have not published our experience, Medical College of Virginia (MCV) Home Care provides a fourth-year elective and teaches some first-, second-, and third-year students during other rotations. There are surely many such unpublished efforts. Additional reports have been found in the Teachers' Section posters at the American Geriatrics Society meeting over the past 5 years. This has been a forum for sharing innovative approaches to geriatric education. Typically, 20 or 30 posters are shown and several mention home care. Most of these programs are electives, or "selectives," where student choose one of several geriatrics experiences. Programs that specifically include home care for medical students are discussed below. Unless otherwise annotated, these programs are described in the abstracts from the annual meetings of the American Geriatrics Society, published in the *Journal of the American Geriatrics Society* in each of the past 5 years.

A 3-week selective is offered to 72 third-year students at Albert Einstein and Montefiore Medical Center in New York, and one of the clinical sites is home care. The University of South Florida has an ambulatory fourth-year elective on end-of-life care, with home visits to 13 terminally ill patients per student. Stanford's program includes 12 fourth-year students on elective who make some house calls. At SUNY, Binghamton, fourth-year students make one required house call during a required month of geriatrics. The University of Kentucky reports a 1-week orientation to geriatric community resources early in the third year, without specifying whether house calls are made. Finally, I mention a unique program run by McMaster University in Toronto: students and residents make 3-day trips with faculty preceptors to an island on Lake Huron, where they provide house calls and other geriatric services.

Obviously, this list captures only selected examples of medical student home care experience. Many students are exposed to home care during community practice rotations and through other "hit-or-miss" mechanisms that are not easily measured. Nor is this an exhaustive tally of formal programs. However, this is a fairly complete list of recently published descriptions. Its brevity suggests that few schools have made home care a substantive focus, and this impression is confirmed by national surveys.

To better define the national picture, in 1982, Nieman explored the connection between family practice and home care by surveying 138 family practice contacts at medical schools, including 16 Canadian schools.[23] Thirty-seven (32%) of 116 responses indicated an undergraduate home care teaching program linked to family practice, and two-thirds of these required some house calls. Nearly half started in the first year. Common learning objectives were observation, social skills, and analysis of families. Medical treatment was included by a minority. The survey was limited to family practice programs and gathered little quantitative data about the home care experience. Still, combined with similar 1979 data,[8] it showed that less than half of U.S. medical schools taught home care, that most programs were elective rather than required, and that medical management of home care patients was not the focus.

Seeking a more current analysis, Steel[10] surveyed medical school deans by telephone in 1994, reaching 95%. Sixty-six of 123 schools reported some home care experience and details were given by 52. Fifteen require home care experience in the first 2 years, and 27 require home care experience in the clinical years. Many require only one house call. Only three schools require students to make six or more house calls during the clinical years and only 18 schools reported lectures on home care. One could argue that deans may lack awareness of small programs on campus, but then by implication those programs not counted would be very small. Thus, things have not changed much in 15 years. Home care does not receive curricular emphasis or support when faced with other priorities and established traditions.

CURRENT HOME CARE EDUCATION FOR RESIDENTS AND GERIATRIC FELLOWS

These more advanced learners require a more discipline-specific, focused curriculum than do medical students. Family practice has historically been the most active specialty for teaching home care. Being focused on comprehensive primary care of patients during all stages of life, this makes sense, and the home care exposure may relate to the greater tendency for practicing family physicians to make house calls, compared with general internists.[24,25]

Family practice is the only discipline whose residency guidelines require home care. Internal medicine now requires a geriatric experience, in reality often a brief rotation embedded in 3 years of training. But internal medicine does not specifically require home care, despite the 1986 position statement by the American College of Physicians[2] that endorses home care capability for internists. Geriatric fellowships, jointly sponsored by family practice and internal medicine, require home care, but the amount of home care experience is not specified and is often modest. Furthermore, although home care is used extensively by many other disciplines, including surgery, obstetrics, pediatrics, and neurology, to name a few, home care is not listed in training guidelines.

EXAMPLES OF RESIDENCY HOME CARE PROGRAMS

I have earlier referred to well-known home care programs at a few centers like Boston University or Johns Hopkins,[26] but there are others. One curriculum was developed at the New Jersey–Rutgers Medical School (now Robert Wood Johnson Medical School) after a statewide survey showed that New Jersey family physicians averaged six house calls per week.[27] The program started in the residents' first year with noon conferences, supplemented by self-instruction materials and self-assessment tools. Second-year residents made house calls, using a decision tree that asked five questions: was transport of the patient impossible? Was the distance realistic? Was the request medically appropriate? Was the request psychosocially appropriate? and did information from another health professional suggest the need for a visit? Another example is the program I started at MCV Home Care in 1987. Early on, we studied our residents, finding favorable attitudes toward the program: 8 of 12 strongly agreed that house calls were valuable educational experiences, and 11 of 12 felt appreciated during visits.[28] Most also agreed that house calls enhanced residents' capabilities and approach to the care of older patients. Following are other examples.

East Boston used house calls made every 8 weeks to teach primary care internal medicine and pediatric residents from Boston City Hospital[29] and found that structured data collection tools and faculty participation helped overcome resistance. Case examples show how house calls enhanced learning not only in the home but at the neighborhood health center. After 3 years, nearly all residents considered the program beneficial.

The University of South Carolina reported over 1,000 house calls by over 100 residents during their introduction to clinical practice.[30] The authors emphasize an initial visit to understand the "get-acquainted, contractual nature" of house calls. Other key features include cross-cultural learning, sharpening observational skills, and timing the teaching house calls to avoid acute illness. Brief exposures were deemed inadequate, and the authors stressed having a series of planned visits with active preceptor supervision. They write: "Not without cost in terms of faculty, resident, and patient time, the end product of home visits—a family physician who is fairly adept at making an efficient and humane home visit—is worth it."

Like medical student education, Teachers' Section posters from the American Geriatrics Society meetings include abstracts on resident education, with some home care. The programs involve several specialties and vary in their intensity, duration, and structure. Following are some examples, again found in the annual meetings abstracts in the *Journal of the American Geriatrics Society.*

Family practice residents at St. Elizabeth Hospital in Ohio have 2 months of geriatrics, including nursing home work, ambulatory assessments, and house calls, plus a syllabus and conference series. Internal medicine residents at the University of Pennsylvania have 1 month of geriatrics. They read relevant clinical material and see several geriatric care settings, including 2 days of home care. Continuing the parade of 1-month rotations is Yale, where geriatrics is required for third-year residents and centers on inpatient rehabilitation and nursing home units, with one required house call. Stanford also has a 1-month block, with a curriculum individualized to learners' needs. Internal medicine residents and geriatric fellows do some home care, which is reserved for more experienced learners. Pittsburgh's Shadyside Hospital internal medicine and family practice programs report a comprehensive approach to geriatric education with two full-time geriatricians and 23 other staff members holding the Geriatric Certificate of Added Qualifications; house calls are part of a 1-month required rotation. Internal medicine residents at the Tucson, Arizona, VA medical center also have a monthlong geriatrics experience, of which 50% is home care, and rate the experience as "superior."

Some programs take a longitudinal approach. The internal medicine program at the Medical Center of Massachusetts in Worcester was redesigned to emphasize primary care, weaving sessions throughout the curriculum, including a series on geriatrics. Residents follow two or three homebound and nursing home patients longitudinally throughout residency. Another longitudinal home care experience is found at the Youville Rehabilitation Hospital program in Cambridge, Massachusetts.

Interdisciplinary team work is the focus at Baylor, where internal medicine residents may choose a 2-month geriatrics elective, one site being Home Based Health Care at the VA hospital. Another mention of interdisciplinary teams comes from SUNY at Buffalo. During a 1-month ambulatory care rotation, internal medicine residents spend one half-day each week on geriatrics. A mobile team with a geriatrician, nurse practitioner, and social worker rotates between clinics, teaching teamwork. Residents must make one house call. Ethnogeriatrics is a focus at the University of California, Irvine, where family medicine residents make house calls with a social worker, then review the cases in an interdisciplinary conference with geriatric fellows and others. Family practice residents at the University of East Carolina also get some home care teaching in the second year.

Finally, a 1-month required geriatrics rotation at Bowman Gray affords internal medicine residents experience in nursing homes, inpatient geriatric consultation, ambulatory geriatric assessment, and home care. In 1993 the Physicians Home Care program was added, with residents following as many as six patients longitudinally. A full-time nurse coordinator organizes the activity, with 119 house calls in the first year. Bowman Gray is mentioned last and highlighted because this program provided my latest physician colleague at MCV Home Care. I doubt I would have been able to recruit her without this preliminary experience.

SURVEY DATA ON RESIDENCY HOME HEALTH CARE TRAINING

Prior to 1994, most nationally representative data about residency home care training were found in family practice surveys. In 1982, Robbins[8] reported that one-fourth of 34 programs taught home care. These data were very general. In the 1980s there were two national studies of home care in family practice residencies.

One was a survey of 375 family practice programs, with 325 responses (86%).[31] Eighty-six percent reported house calls, more than half including nocturnal visits. Hindrances to teaching house calls were: time (36%), finances (27%), inappropriateness for the program (22%), distance (18%), and safety (13%). Program directors agreed that: "home visits are a small but important part of a family physician's practice," "home visits are time-consuming but useful," and "resident education should include information on how to make home visits." The directors disagreed with other attitudes: "Physicians should not make home visits because the tools necessary for diagnosis can be used only in the office," and "Information about functioning obtained on a home visit can be obtained in the office." Most directors also disagreed that "home visits are a poor use of a physician's time." Forty-one percent of programs offered additional curricula on home care. The authors noted that residents early in training benefit from direct faculty supervision and from structured data collection tools. The survey does not quantify home care teaching, whether the residents are required to participate, or the amount of didactic home care instruction.

In 1987, Laguillo surveyed 380 family practice programs,[32] with 282 responses (74%). During 3 years of residency, the hours dedicated to geriatrics numbered between 200 and 400 in half of the programs, with a third using less than 200 hours and 15% dedicating over 400 hours. Less than 10% of geriatric teaching time focused on home care. A third of the programs taught longitudinal management of home care patients. Home care was felt to have most value in teaching continuity of care, work with multidisciplinary teams, and cost containment. Resident perception of home care experiences was thought generally favorable.

The authors emphasize longitudinal, continuity-oriented experiences and consider home care particularly suited to learning these concepts:

> Principles of team management and interdisciplinary and multidisciplinary approach to health care, impact of the social environment on health and disease, implementation of rehabilitation protocols, appropriate use of community-based support systems for the elderly, home assessment of the functional status of the elderly, risk analysis and accident prevention, recognition of the role of the caregiver and the stressors involved in the patient-caregiver relation at home, the role of intermediate care of the recently acutely ill patient, and the importance of discharge planning and its implementation . . . and to learn about family interviewing skills, assessment of family dynamics and its implications for care of the elderly, and the ability to obtain a holistic view of the aged within the context of their sociocultural milieu.

Recently, the Task Force on Geriatric Medicine of the Society of General Internal Medicine (SGIM) studied geriatric education in all U.S. family practice and internal medicine residencies. Separate surveys were conducted for acute care, ambulatory care, nursing home care, and home care, each time dividing geriatric educational goals into three domains: knowledge, attitudes, and skills.[11] This project defined curricular elements best taught in each venue and which educational methods work best.

In 1994 the SGIM task force mailed 796 surveys to program directors regarding home care education, with 504 responses (63%) evenly divided by specialty. Most family practice residents (92%) make some house calls, usually in a longitudinal model, compared with 33% of internal medicine residents whose home care experience comes in block rotations or brief, one-time exposures. Program directors view home care as important, yet the primary reported barrier to teaching home care is limited faculty time, reinforcing the directors' stated view that competing priorities are a problem. Overall, the investment in home care training is not impressive. Most internal medicine residents reportedly receive less than 10 hours of teaching on home care, spread over 3 years; family practice programs cluster between 10 and 25 hours. For perspective, this would be equivalent to 1 day and night of inpatient hospital work. Thus, though attitudes are generally supportive, these programs have far to go.

The SGIM task force used the survey data to create guidelines for geriatric curriculum planning in nursing homes, acute care, home care, and ambulatory care. The nursing home guidelines are a prototype, addressing both structure and content.[33] Content recommendations come from prioritized rankings of several dozen topics. The SGIM geriatric home care curriculum guidelines are now available. The basic approach to teaching home care has not changed; many of the SGIM recommendations echo those of Laguillo with respect to longitudinal care management, functional status, and psychosocial and caregiver support issues. But the new guidelines are more specific about medical content and program structure.

PERSONAL OBSERVATIONS ON PREPARING YOUNG PHYSICIANS FOR HOME CARE

First, I am encouraged. Slowly, home care is entering medical school and postgraduate curricula. Counterbalancing this optimism is awareness of the very small role home care still plays, even where it is better developed and championed. A discouraging number of programs require only one house call. Second, some approaches are better than others. Practice-based family practice programs often build longitudinal home care into the weekly routine, but many residencies use blocks. Blocks are expeditious and fit the rotational structure of many residencies. However, blocks diminish continuity and lessen the chances to reinforce lessons. Some reinforcement is critical. Third, the success of many home care teaching programs hinges on a few key individuals. We urgently need more faculty development.

When teaching residents home care, there are some principles one must follow. First, residents need to go into homes, crossing the threshold, overcoming inertia and fear of the unfamiliar, and "taking the plunge." Next is a sense of value and responsibility. Residents need to feel that their work is worthwhile and to have some autonomy in making patient care decisions. Simply watching others work, or "sitting in" briefly in the middle of a long course of home care has less value. To accomplish these objectives, residents require role models and active instruction during home care work. It is hard to persuade residents to make house calls if their teachers do not make house calls. Residents are sometimes viewed as load-bearing clinical providers, this being part of the price of their education.

Only if there is active teaching will house calls be accepted. Burton[24] writes, "sophisticated judgement is necessary to care for very ill patients at home, and the housecall should be performed by more advanced resident physicians and taught by the best general physicians."

Throughout education, one certain key to success is inspiring teachers. Even unpleasant topics can be made interesting by the right teacher. Home care providers are typically fierce advocates and dedicated clinicians; many, but not all, are also skillful teachers. Home care education involves not only advocacy but recognizing the needs of the students and creating a specific curriculum that imparts knowledge and skill. The cadre of effective home care teachers and teaching programs is very small, so the future of home care depends on finding more such individuals and attracting them to this field. Curricula likewise must accommodate students headed for subspecialized areas of medical practice, whose relationship to home care will be different from that of generalists.

Developing and sheltering faculty is also vital. Over the years, MCV Home Care has been fairly successful, providing a low-intensity, longitudinal experience for primary care residents. Yet we have periodically lost key faculty, and it has sometimes been a struggle to keep our small program healthy from both a clinical and an educational viewpoint. House calls do not yield sufficient revenue to shield faculty from fiscal pressures, and burnout is common for faculty who have home care as a major responsibility. These factors make recruitment and retention challenging. I have explored distributing home care teaching across the large faculty group in general medicine and geriatrics who have many strengths but make very few house calls. Other commitments dominate, whether these involve health services research, specialized programs for HIV-infected patients, or traditional internal medicine primary care practice and teaching. Thus, they do no share the home care teaching load, and home care remains separate, self-contained, and vulnerable. Our story is not unique.

Home care teachers must realize that residents are pulled away from other high-intensity responsibilities to work in ambulatory care, nursing homes, and home care. Their outpatient work has suffered from a lower sense of urgency. Care of "sick" inpatients, supervising interns, and preparing for future board exams are their priorities. Home care must become more valuable in their eyes. The activity must use and refine medical skills, and the pressure to return to the wards must be lessened, calling for help from residency directors.

Safety bears further mention. Many residents are anxious about personal safety during house calls, particularly in urban or very isolated rural settings. Understandably, this issue is especially troublesome to women. Considering the safety record of other home care professionals, these fears are sometimes exaggerated or uninformed, but they are real and must be respected.

No discussion of residency home care teaching programs would be complete without mentioning funding. Aside from the meager clinical income from house calls, funding for home care education can come through several avenues. Grants are the most obvious but tend to be small and transient. Another strategy, underutilized, is linking home care education to home health agency care. Medicare rules (section 206.5) state: "Home health services include the medical services of interns and residents-in-training under an approved hospital teaching program if the agency has an affiliation with or is under common control of a hospital providing such medical services." Thus, home health agencies can be reimbursed for residents' house calls. Efforts organized through home health agencies still require medical faculty to inspire, guide, and teach the students, plus support from residency directors.

A larger issue is implied by the Medicare "pass-through" funds given to teaching hospitals to support the cost of postgraduate training. As Medicare increasingly emphasizes home care in place of hospital care, it seems logical that proportionately more residency funding will follow the clinical emphasis, and programs that respond to the transformation may be rewarded. Private payers will likewise be investing in medical education, and they will need to reminded about the importance of home care.

The long-term impact of home care teaching efforts is also largely unknown. Talking with residency graduates suggests that they retain what they learned and continue to make house calls, albeit infrequently. Colleagues at other teaching home care programs also tell success stories, but this area requires formal study.

A new challenge now faces home care faculty in residency programs, along with a new opportunity. Residencies are under great pressure to shift teaching into outpatient settings. Although home care epitomizes outpatient primary care, the emphasis is now on office-based practice. This is the challenge.

Here is the opportunity. Residency should mirror population needs and community practice demands, and it is time for home care advocates to trumpet their value. The increasing elderly population, the explosion of physician-ordered home care services, and the shift away from hospital care constitute a mandate. Home care's central role in the continuum of services must be recognized. It is time for strong advocacy and strategic, proactive program development.

HOME CARE EDUCATION FOR POSTGRADUATE PHYSICIANS AND OTHER PROFESSIONALS

Information on fellowship home care teaching is even less available than information about undergraduate and resident programs. The few geriatric fellows are primarily being groomed for academic or management roles. Their training occurs primarily at university programs, many linked to VA medical centers. The amount and quality of home care experience for geriatric fellows varies, but nursing homes clearly dominate both long-term care research and clinical education. These fellowship graduates will become future leaders, so we can only hope that their exposure to home care is sufficient to promote wise future policies.

Let us look away from physicians for a moment because home care needs working teams of physicians and other professionals. Thus, the education of nurses, physical therapists, social workers, and others who will fill home care roles should include experiences to prepare them for working partnerships with home care physicians. There is room for improvement, judging by some of the calls I receive from other home care workers. Physicians need to know more about home care and about home health agency operations (see below), but agency personnel also need more understanding of physicians' needs and issues. This interface needs much work, as discussed in chapter 3. Home care physicians have much to offer as educators.

CONTINUING EDUCATION FOR PRACTICING PHYSICIANS

There is abundant evidence that many practicing physicians could benefit from more education about home care. Whether looking at studies of hospital care that show unrecognized needs for home care among discharged patients,[34] physician surveys, or home health agency surveys, the message is clear. In the 1990 national physician survey, among physicians who made few home health agency referrals, only 59% agreed with the item "I have sufficient knowledge of community services to personally plan or deliver home health care." Even among physicians who made at least 48 annual referrals to home health agencies, averaging 95 referrals, 15% considered their knowledge of community services insufficient. Knowledge of community resources remained a significant predictor of home care referrals in a multivariable analysis that included numerous physician and practice characteristics.[35]

The ultimate cure for this problem will come through changing undergraduate and graduate education, but continuing medical education is needed now. One example of how this can be accomplished is a program that Dr. Joanne Schwartzberg established with support from the American Medical Association and the Agency on Aging. Relying on opinion leaders in local medical associations, Dr. Schwartzberg and her collaborators developed a case-based workshop that has been given in several states and serves as a model for future efforts. Another example is the Home Health Agency Medical Director Training Workshop series now being offered by the American Academy of Home Care Physicians.

EDUCATING THE PUBLIC

One frustration for all home care professionals is that the general public has limited understanding of the benefits and the limitations of home care. On one hand, I have seen people suffer because they did not recognize their eligibility for home care or because they refused services for reasons of pride, privacy, or general mistrust. I have also spent much time and energy explaining the limits of home care coverage to desperate people, as have my colleagues in other home health professions. This isn't rewarding or cost-effective. The more that people know about home care, the easier delivering home care will be.

From this educated public will also come future professionals, again having personal memories of physicians making house calls. Finally, political pressure to support home care derives from the people in this democracy. If people understand home care, want more home care, and voice their desire, more home care will eventually follow. Physicians should set a visible example and speak out publicly for home care when opportunities arise.

WHAT IS AHEAD FOR MEDICAL EDUCATION

The strength of the movement to change medical education and invigo-rate primary care is shown in the September 7, 1994, *Journal of the American Medical Association*, dedicated exclusively to medical educa-tion. This is an excellent review of key issues, as is the April 1994 sup-plement to the *Journal of General Internal Medicine*, on the education of general internists. The papers are broad in scope, with little specific men-tion of home care, yet they emphasize tailoring medical education to the needs of populations and communities. The forces behind the change in strategies have been clearly and repeatedly expressed, along with concern about the role of academic centers.[36–38] Federman wrote:[39]

> The flowering of complex surgery, antibiotics, cancer chemotherapy, and coronary and intensive care created an endlessly fascinating world in which patient care, medical education, and clinical research could all thrive simultaneously. But the recent evolution of the university teach-ing hospital has become skewed. It is more than ever a center of applied pathophysiology, but less and less a place where patients can rest, recu-perate, or die, and it is correspondingly a less useful site for future doc-tors to learn basic clinical skills.

Some answers to such challenges are now appearing. Countering the trend for medical students to avoid primary care fields[40] are proactive visions about the excitement of primary care internal medicine,[41] until recently a field often chosen by physicians seeking coveted subspecial-ized practices. Meanwhile, according to two recognized authorities, sub-specialists will have four roles: as consultants to generalists and their patients, as providers of advanced clinical care for patients with highly complex problems, as scholars and educators, and as physician scientists involved in research.[42]

The chairman of medicine at UCLA recently described restructuring the internal medicine program: general internal medicine clinician-edu-cators would be paid 10% *more* than invasive cardiologists and other sub-specialists. Subspecialty training would produce a few academicians rather than many clinicians, and general internists' training would produce broadly competent individuals capable of functioning with less subspe-cialist support. Among 25 new generalist faculty members would be sev-eral geriatricians.[43] Looking eastward, SUNY at Buffalo proposes an "academic health center without walls" concept.[44] The medical education literature is now flooded with such issues.

This transformation has implications for home care education. Being principally a generalist activity centered on community needs, home care should witness a renaissance in medical education, paralleling the expansion of home care practice. Simultaneously, subspecialists may have new incentives to support the home care practices of generalist colleagues, and there may be more specialty consultation at home. As inefficient as it seems to transport a highly trained subspecialist to a patient's home, the alternative cost of transporting the immobile patient may be even greater. Care delivery systems accepting financial risk may encourage subspecialists to make rounds in the community.

Anticipating this movement, medical schools are changing recruitment strategies and selection criteria. They are building programs to nourish humanism, and they are expanding areas outside the traditional biomedical menu of curricular content. I have found house calls an excellent means to help people retain or rediscover compassion and humanistic attributes. Home care has other unique features as a learning experience, one of which is an emphasis on awareness of the surroundings. This involves a form of learning different from the scientific empiricism that has fostered medical progress in the past century. Neither approach is necessarily superior, and both have their place. In home care the learning is more experiential, which is the preferred learning process for many generalist clinicians.

Perhaps even seeing a videotape or a live video transmission of a familiar case, not just an abstract case "off the shelf," would render home care lessons vital and relevant because we cannot currently expect all hospital-based medical students to make house calls. There is an unlimited supply of cases in which home care offers a compelling contrast to the inpatient experience. Home care education needs new ideas as well as more champions and more teachers.

REFERENCES

1. Vladeck BC. From the Health Care Financing Administration: The Medicare Home Health Initiative. *JAMA*. 1994; 271:1566.
2. Health and Public Policy Committee of the American College of Physicians. Home health care. *Ann Intern Med*. 1986; 105:454–460.

3. Council on Scientific Affairs of the American Medical Association. Educating physicians in home health care. *JAMA.* 1991; 265:769–771.

4. American Geriatrics Society Public Policy Committee. Home care and home care reimbursement. *J Am Geriatr Soc.* 1989; 37:1065–1066.

5. Beall C, Baumhover LA, Simpson JA, Pieroni RE. Teaching geriatric medicine: Residents' perceptions of barriers and stereotypes. *Gerontol Geriatr Educ.* 1991; 11(3):85–95.

6. Martini CJM, Veloski JJ, Barzansky B, Xu G, Fields SK. Medical schools and student characteristics that influence choosing a generalist career. *JAMA.* 1994; 272:661–668.

7. Coccaro EF, Miles AM. The attitudinal impact of training in gerontology/ geriatrics in medical school: A review of the literature and perspective. *J Am Geriatr Soc.* 1984; 32:762–768.

8. Robbins AS, Vivell S, Beck JC. A study of geriatric training programs in the United States. *J Med Educ.* 1982; 57:79–86.

9. Schwartzberg JG. Home care education for physicians. *Caring.* May 1992; 18–24.

10. Steel K, Musliner MC, Boling P. Medical schools and home care. *N Engl J Med.* 1994; 331:1098–1099.

11. Boling PA. Paper presented at the annual meeting of the American Geriatrics Society. May 1995.

12. Wener S, Foley C, Jaffe A. Three years of a required geriatrics module for third-year medical students. *Academic Medicine.* 1991; 66(5):292–294.

13. Olson E, Libow L, Tideiksaar R, Bodin L, Hsu MA. Long term effects of a mandatory fourth year medical student rotation in geriatric medicine. *J Am Geriatr Soc.* 1991; 39(8):A83. Abstract.

14. Glanos AN, Cohen HJ, Jackson TW. Medical education in geriatrics: The lasting impact of the aging game. *J Am Geriatr Soc.* 1991; 39(8):A41. Abstract.

15. McCahan JF, Bissonette AM, DiRusso BA. A house call teaching program for fourth-year medical students. *J Med Educ.* 1983; 58:349–351.

16. Keenan JM, Bland CJ, Webster L, Myers S. The home care practice and attitudes of Minnesota family physicians. *J Am Geriatr Soc.* 1991; 39:1100–1104.

17. Keenan JM, Hepburn KW, Ripsin CM, Webster L, Bland CJ. A survey of home care agencies' perceptions of physicians behaviors. *Family Medicine.* 1992; 24(2):142–144.

18. Steel K. Physician-directed long-term home health care for the elderly: A century-long experience. *J Am Geriatr Soc.* 1987; 35:264–268.

19. Birenbaum A, Aronson M, Seiffer S. Training medical students to appreciate the special problems of the elderly. *Gerontologist.* 1979; 19:575–579.

20. Billings JA, Coles R, Reiser SJ, Stoeckle JD. A seminar in "plain doctoring." *J Med Educ.* 1985; 60:855–859.

21. Page AEK, Walker-Bartnick L, Taler GA, Snow DA, Wertheimer DS, Al-

Ibrahim MS. A program to teach house calls for the elderly to fourth year medical students. *J Med Educ.* 1988; 63:51–58.

22. Sankar A, Becker SL. The home as a site for teaching gerontology and chronic illness. *J Med Educ.* 1985; 60:308–313.

23. Nieman LZ, Jones JG. Family medicine home visit programs in U.S. and Canadian medical schools. *J Med Educ.* 1983; 58:934–940.

24. Boling PA, Retchin SM, Ellis J, Pancoast SA. The influence of physician specialty on housecalls. *Arch Intern Med.* 1990; 150:2333–2337.

25. Keenan JM, Boling PA, Schwartzberg JG, Olson L, Schneiderman M, McCaffrey DJ, Ripsin CM. A National Survey of the Home Visiting Practice and Attitudes of Family Physicians and Internists. *Arch Intern Med.* 1992; 152:2025–2032.

26. Burton JR. The house call: An important service for the frail elderly. *J Am Geriatr Soc.* 1985; 33(4):291–293.

27. Warburton SW, Sadler GR. House call training in the family practice curriculum. *J Med Educ.* 1977; 52:768–770.

28. Boling PA, Buchsbaum DG, Pancoast SA, Buchanan RG. Primary care internal medicine residents' responses to a continuity-oriented longitudinal home-visit experience. *Teaching and Learning in Medicine.* 1990; 2(1):34–37.

29. Young R, Freiberg E, Stringham P. The home visit in the multidisciplinary teaching of primary care physicians. *J Med Educ.* 1981; 56:341–346.

30. Guy LJ, Schuman SH. Home visits as curriculum. *J Fam Pract.* 1982; 14(1):26–27.

31. Graham AV, Krick JP. Family home assessment in family practice residency programs. *J Fam Pract.* 1981; 13(2):217–221.

32. Laguillo E. Home care services as teaching sites for geriatrics in family medicine residencies. *J Med Educ.* 1988; 63(9):667–674.

33. Counsell SR, Katz PR, Karuza J, Sullivan GM. Resident Training in nursing home care: Survey of successful educational strategies. *J Am Geriatr Soc.* 1994; 42:1193–1199.

34. Jones EW, Densen PM, Brown SD. Post hospital needs of elderly people at home: Findings from an eight-month follow-up study. *Health Serv Res.* 1989; 24:643–664.

35. Boling PA, Keenan JM, Schwartzberg JS, Retchin SM, Olson L, Schneiderman M. Reported home health agency referrals by internists and family physicians. *J Am Geriatr Soc.* 1992; 40:1241–1249.

36. Rosenblatt RA, Whitcomb ME Cullen TJ, Lishner DM, Hart LG. The effect of federal grants on medical schools' production of primary care physicians. *Am J Public Health.* 1993; 83:322–328.

37. Petersdorf RG. Commentary: Primary care-medical students' unpopular choice. *Am J Public Health.* 1993; 83:328–330.

38. Blumenthal D, Meyer GS. The future of the academic medical center under health care reform. *N Engl J Med.* 1993; 329:1812–1814.

39. Federman DD. Medical education in outpatient settings. *N Engl J Med.* 1989; 320:1536–1537.
40. Geiger HJ. Why don't medical students choose primary care? *Am J Public Health.* 1993; 83:315–316.
41. Lipkin M, Levinson W, Barker R, Kern D, Burke W, Noble J, Wartman S, Delbanco TL. Primary care internal medicine: A challenging career choice for the 1990s. *Ann Intern Med.* 1990; 112:371–378.
42. Kimball HR, Bennett JC. Training the future internal medicine subspecialist. *Am J Med.* 1994; 96:559–561.
43. Fogelman AM. Strategies for training generalists and subspecialists. *Ann Intern Med.* 1994; 120:579–583.
44. Naughton J, Vana JE. The academic health center and the healthy community. *Am J Public Health.* 1994; 84:1071–1076.

CHAPTER 12

Physician and Professional Provider Compensation in Home Health Care

I nadequate physician compensation for house calls and home care management is a major factor in the reluctance of many physicians to be more actively involved.[1-6] I state this boldly, knowing that health care spending is over $3 billion per day and that physicians are widely considered both affluent and overly concerned with their own financial self-interest.

BASICS OF MEDICARE PHYSICIAN PAYMENT AND THE COST OF HOUSE CALLS

Summarized below are the CPT descriptions for house calls. When providers bill Part B of Medicare, they use CPT codes from the manual *Current Procedural Terminology* to indicate what services(s) they provided. A payment schedule built around these codes determines compensation. The CPT code descriptions specifically require certain elements for a given service, such as taking a history, but other activities are "bundled," such as when a patient is weighed or has blood drawn. Counseling patients or families and coordinating home care is bundled with house calls in all but very complex cases.

> 99341 (new patient) and 99351 (established patient): Home visit; problem-focused history; problem focused exam; medical decision-making is straightforward or of low complexity; for established patients if stable, recovering or improving.
>
> 99342 (new patient) and 99352 (established patient): Home visit; expanded problem-focused history; expanded problem-focused exam; medical decision-making of moderate complexity; for established patients responding inadequately to treatment or with a minor complication.
>
> 99343 (new patient) and 99353 (established patient): Home visit with detailed history; detailed exam; medical decision-making of high complexity; for established patients if unstable or with significant complications or new problems.
>
> For all house calls, care coordination and family counseling as appropriate are considered part of the service.

Shown in Table 12.1 are Medicare's current allowable payments for house calls in my region. Recall here from chapter 10 that house calls consumed from 15 (bare minimum) to 90 minutes or more in my survey of Virginia physicians, averaging 52 minutes, including travel. In Adelman's national survey most house calls fell into the 20- to 40-minute category (56%), or the 40- to 60-minute category (29%), and travel time was not mentioned. The Medical College of Virginia (MCV) Home Care staff average 1 hour, including travel, for a mixture of new and established patients. Office overhead follows most physicians who make house calls, accumulating during time spent driving and during subsequent care management.

Virginia Medicaid payments for house calls are shown in Table 12.2. Table 12.3 demonstrates national Medicare house call services and payments in recent years. And while private carriers are more generous, home care payment policies vary. An example from a large private payer in my area is shown in Table 12.4.

George Taler argues cogently that the economic hardship of carrying office overhead on house calls can be blunted by reducing office support while physicians make house calls and by hiring a home care coordinator. These are feasible strategies in offices heavily committed to home care, but even then they do not eradicate the fiscal hardship.

TABLE 12.1 1996 Medicare House Call Fee Schedule; Richmond, VA

New patients	Par fee $ allow*	Established patients	Par fee $ allow*
99341	57.07	99351	45.06
99342	71.89	99352	56.82 (most common service)
99343	92.36	99353	68.94

* Allowable fee for participating physicians; 80% is paid by Medicare, with a 20% patient co-payment

TABLE 12.2 1996 Virginia Medicaid House Call Fee Schedule

CPT code	Pays ($)	CPT code	Pays ($)
99341	30.00	99351	10.00
99342	33.60	99352	27.50 (most common service)
99343	35.15	99353	34.05

Consider the operation of a typical office practice. Operating costs, excluding physician salary, of a self-employed physician in 1992 included office cost (25%), professional staff (37%), medical supplies (10%) and equipment (4%), liability insurance (7%), and "other" (19%), totaling $179,000.[7] If the office physician made house calls 1 half-day per week, most of this overhead would remain. Net income was about 45% of gross income for general practice and family physicians in 1989, about 48% for pediatricians, 50% for general internists, and 50% to 60% for most specialists.[8]

Office visit time is another useful point of reference. Family physician office visits run as follows: 6–10 minutes (28%), 11–15 minutes (30%), and 16–30 minutes (23%). Only 6% of encounters take more than 30 minutes.[9] Corresponding data for internists are 6–10 minutes (20%), 11–15 minutes (39%), 16–30 minutes (27%), and over 30 minutes (7%).[10] Internists spend 27 hours per week in office settings, and family physicians spend 35 hours. Both disciplines report nearly 50 hours per week of direct patient care and about 55 weekly hours of total patient care work. These disciplines respectively see 112 and 146 patients per week.[11]

TABLE 12.3 Medicare House Call Payments

CPT code	1992 No. of services	Avg.($) paid	1993 No. of services	Avg.($) paid	1994 No. of services	Avg.($) paid	1995 No. of services	Avg.($) paid
99341	51,003	42	61,383	46	67,443	51	68,621	58
99342	62,222	51	62,903	57	67,288	64	64,764	74
99343	34,185	65	43,712	71	48,476	81	50,675	93
99351	374,329	34	422,133	37	447,531	41	436,041	45
99352	494,368	43	539,686	47	586,570	54	590,115	58
99353	230,230	53	276,688	57	340,050	64	350,603	72

Source: Health Care Financing Administration.

TABLE 12.4 A Richmond, VA Private Payer's 1996 House Call Fee Schedule (Preferred Provider Network)

CPT code	Payment ($)	CPT code	Payment ($)
99341	65.00	99351	48.00
99342	82.00	99352	66.00
99343	107.00	99353	83.00

REVENUE NEEDED TO SUPPORT HOUSE CALLS

Having looked at costs, the next issue is the revenue needed to support physician salaries and overhead. Revenue derives from many sources, including fee-for-service payments, ancillary services like laboratory testing, and capitation contracts. Ancillary services are often an important revenue source, one currently difficult to obtain in home care.

Suppose a physician makes house calls 1 half-day per week. If the physician's salary is $100,000 and overhead consumes 55% of gross income, the physician must generate $222,000, with $122,000 going to overhead. Given 250 working days per year, gross income would average $440 per half-day, with $200 going to net and $240 going to overhead. On average, five house calls fill a half-day (8 to 12:30 or 1 to 5:30). Under these assumptions, the physician would need $88 per average house call, including travel but not the additional care management time that is often substantial.

When surveyed, physicians arrive at remarkably similar figures. We asked a national sample of clinically active family physicians and internists (1,161 responses) how much they charged for a 45–60-minute house call, including travel, and how much payment they would need to make such house calls financially feasible.[3] They reported mean charges of $60, median charges of $50, and a range from $18 to $220. Estimated payments to make house calls feasible were $113 (mean) and $100 (median), ranging from $10 to $600. Sixteen percent were between $50 and $60, and 35% sought $120 or more. Only 4% would accept under $50. About half of the respondents made house calls.

My 1988 statewide survey of Virginia primary care physicians yielded comparable numbers.[4] Respondents estimated "fair payment for a 45-minute home visit" as follows: general internal medicine ($81), family practice ($72), general practice ($56), and subspecialized internists ($98). For comparison, office visit charges were as follows: general internists ($31), family physicians ($25), general practitioners ($24), and subspecialists ($33).

Thus, Medicare's house call payments are well below cost, and they are a financial disincentive. Now contrast Medicare house call payments with Medicare payments for other home care services. Shown in Table 12.5 are 1996 Medicare cost limits for my region that define the value accorded these common services. Home health agencies bear large administrative costs, created largely by the need to comply with detailed federal regulations governing home health agencies. However, physicians with offices practices also spend at least 50% to 60% of gross income on overhead.

Payment for professional provider home care work would be another important subject for practice managers. As discussed in chapter 3, Medicare allows reimbursement for professional provider house calls only in federally designated Health Manpower Shortage areas. Medicaid gives states the option of paying for professional provider house calls without restricting the service to manpower shortage areas, but Medicaid pays very little per service. Because there are powerful arguments for encouraging home care work by professional providers, one can only hope that federal payment policy for house calls will follow the example of nursing home care, where professional provider visits are allowable.

Given frail homebound patients, the caseload for an experienced home

TABLE 12.5 1996 Medicare Home Health Agency Cost Limits Richmond, VA

Home health agency service	Labor ($)	Nonlabor ($)	Medicare total cost limit ($)
Home nursing visit	76.57	21.62	98.19
Home physical therapy visit	83.84	23.99	107.43
Home social work visit	110.59	31.46	142.05

care nurse practitioner or physician assistant is about 40 to 50. With a salary of $45,000 or $50,000 in my region, plus 26% for benefits, and projecting about 20 home visits per week for a full-time home care nurse practitioner,[12] the needed payment per house call would be $65 plus overhead. As these are full-time home care providers, the $65 figure includes care management work but does not include secretarial support, supplies, billing, malpractice coverage, and travel expenses (overhead).

Let us finally consider care (or case) management work, the continuing effort before and after the direct patient contact that consumes a lot of time when caring for complex homebound patients. Some home care patients require little care management, but the others challenge physicians and their professional associates. A time-motion study of the Rochester Home Care Team that served medically ill patients found care management occupying 40% of all physician and nurse practitioner time.[13] Travel consumed 20% and direct patient contact involved 40%. Care management included phone contact with patients and families (4% of work), phone contact with other professionals (7%), record writing (10%), care conferences (5%), and miscellaneous other nontelephone care coordination (13%). Direct contact in the home was 23% of physician effort, and inpatient care used 15%. Patient contact time during house calls averaged 39 minutes for physicians and 49 minutes for nurse practitioners.

Compared with office practice, there are two major distinctions. First, the likelihood that home care patients will need active support between direct encounters is far higher. Second, office patients with complex needs can visit the office more often, supporting the provider's time through visit fees. The immobility of the homebound limits this option, and a compensatory increase in house call frequency simply increases the deficit, because of poor house call reimbursement.

RECENT CHANGES IN PHYSICIAN PAYMENTS

The need to systematically revise physician payment resulted in the Resource Based Relative Value Scale (RBRVS), planned in the 1980s as a method for fairly apportioning Medicare physician payments. Using a standardized reference unit, the RVU (relative value unit), the RBRVS assigns values to three elements of each service: physician work (before, during, and after direct contact); specialty-specific practice costs, adjusted regionally; and opportunity costs for physician training.[14] This approach was intended to create a payment schedule similar to one that would evolve under free market conditions. Values were assigned after reviews of published data and interviews of practitioners by a selected expert panel for each discipline. This complex analysis captured some of the differences between specialties and services. For example, 1983 family physician practice costs were estimated to be 48% of gross revenues, compared with 22% for psychiatrists.[15]

Gradual implementation of the RBRVS fee schedule was expected to increase the compensation for evaluation and management (cognitive) services, compared with procedural services.[16] Looking back, the RBRVS architects found that the fee schedule has not fulfilled expectations.[17] If all physicians were paid according to 1992 charges, pediatricians' income would have been $71,000; family physicians' income, $81,000; and general internists' income, $127,000, compared with invasive cardiologists at $930,000 and thoracic surgeons at $934,000. However, if payments followed the 1992 RBRVS schedule, respective incomes would have been $35,000, $40,000, $44,000, $221,000, and $241,000. The authors noted two main problems: underestimation of practice costs when the RBRVS schedule was created and using historical charges to define practice costs, disproportionately favoring procedural services for which practice costs had been inflated. The subsequent history of adjustments to the RBRVS reveals the logistic and political challenges encountered when one makes major changes in payments of over $200 billion to 600,000 highly paid professionals.

Advocacy is one critical factor, as house calls demonstrate. The newly formed American Academy of Home Care Physicians has now joined the debate, proposing an increase in house call value and leading a national review of house call work. Previously, unlike more common physician services, house calls were never directly studied; work and practice expense values were simply assigned. Therefore, in 1995, as part of a national 5-year review of physician payment, hundreds of physicians were surveyed regarding house call work. Compared with office visits, house call patients tend to have more complex medical needs, and house calls require substantially more time and work in evaluating functional status, social support, and home environments, plus much caregiver counseling. Care management, before and after the visit, also tends to be greater.

In April 1996 these arguments were accepted by the American Medical Association's Resource Update Committee (RUC), a 23-member body with national representation from many specialties that is charged with overseeing fair assignment of work values across all physician services. The RUC also recognized that there are no appropriate codes for the most complex house calls and recommended that these be created. Another matter, yet to be addressed, is that house calls were excluded from the 1993 proposal to allow payment on special modifier codes used when billing Medicare for unusually complex and time-consuming cases in offices, hospitals, and nursing homes.

Recent RBRVS history also highlights the importance of accurately measuring practice costs, which is particularly relevant to home care. Compared with office visits, driving time adds expense, and for most physicians house calls carry fixed overhead costs from their office practices, such as rent or mortgage, utilities, staff salaries, upkeep, and supplies, that must be covered. House call practice expense is being studied in 1996. A corollary concern may soon emerge, related to differences in practice expense between full-time home care physicians and those who are primarily office-based. As house call practice becomes a proportionately larger share of a given physician's total work, overhead should fall. Fee schedules may ultimately need to be adjusted, and home care specialists may become a separate class of providers.

The latest revisions in the RBRVS fee schedule may accord house calls some of the largest payment increases of any Medicare services. However, house call payment started so low that reimbursement is still below cost for most physicians. The Physician Payment Review Commission noted the declining frequency of housecalls and the impact of low reimbursement in their 1994 report to Congress,[18] highlighting the importance of this issue, as follows.

> Home visits represent only a minuscule portion of total EM services. Physicians on average provide less than one home visit for every 100

office visits billed to Medicare, and home visits account for less than 0.2 percent of Medicare physician' services payments.

Home visits may nonetheless be of significant interest on several counts. First, the homebound represent perhaps one of the most vulnerable Medicare populations. Declines in primary care services to this population might therefore merit more attention than would changes in services provided to other Medicare beneficiaries. Second, as noted home visit services take a considerable amount of physician time, but are relatively poorly paid. In 1992, Medicare paid $43 for the average physician home visit, versus $32 for the average office visit. The $11 fee difference seems unlikely to compensate for the additional time and inconvenience involved. Advisers to the Commission have suggested that the combination of time and low hourly remuneration along with financial pressures on providers' practices might make home visits a service that is curtailed by providers.

CARE PLAN OVERSIGHT (CPO)

As seen in earlier chapters, most paid home health care is delivered by home health agencies with physician guidance. Sometimes this physician work is considerable. Recently, the Health Care Financing Administration (HCFA) endorsed greater physician involvement in home care and agreed to further compensate physicians for care management in selected home care cases. First surfacing in 1993 as a proposal to pay for high-tech cases, care plan oversight (CPO) payment[19] became available in January 1995. Based on 1.63 RVUs, or about $50, this payment is allowed in cases that consume 30 minutes or more of physician time spent on home care medical decision making and record review each month for Medicare patients concurrently receiving skilled services from a certified home health agency. The physician must also have seen the patient within 6 months' time. CPO payment in appropriate cases and with patient notification regarding co-payments was endorsed by the National Association for Home Care, which represents home health agency concerns. Late in 1995 the CPO work value was increased to 1.73 RVUs.

Although CPO payment is an important step, it is limited. For one thing, CPO excludes most home care cases, those that don't reach the 30-minute threshold; yet these have a large cumulative impact. At MCV

Home Care, about 30% of a medically ill, chronically homebound population receive Medicare skilled home health care in any given month. Many of these require less than 30 minutes of care management. Ten percent or less of our cases qualify for CPO payment each month. If 10% of homebound patients qualified for CPO and we applied this figure to 1990 national survey data, where office-based physicians reported following 20 homebound patients, those physicians would have two cases eligible for CPO payment each month. However, such physicians might well have 10 other active home care patients, each needing 15 minutes per month. Together, they would take 2.5 hours, worth $250 of physician time. Recall, then, that the 1990 national survey found internists and family physicians reporting over 3 hours per *week* for home care management.[20] A significant uncompensated burden remains.

Part of this burden is from time spent counseling patients and caregivers by phone, which MCV Home Care staff find very time-consuming. Work with caregivers is excluded by CPO policy. CPO further excludes patients who are not receiving skilled home health agency services. Five or ten percent of MCV Home Care patients require extensive care management despite being "too stable" for medical skilled home health agency care. These are cases for which informal caregivers provide the equivalent of skilled care, cases with major neuropsychiatric components, and complex social situations. Home care patients have unpredictably changing courses. They often require physician effort, particularly through telephone conversations with caregivers and "curbside consults" with other professionals, long after Medicare home health agency care, designed for acute and postacute illness, has ended.

For example, a demented patient caused her two sons to fight, resulting in broken bones. I was on the phone with one of them every few days about her strange behavior or their family conflict, and I helped form the ultimate plan for her to enter a nursing home. Yet she had no indication for home health agency care. For years another woman with Alzheimer's disease has lived with her emotionally labile but dedicated daughter. The caregiver and family are conflicted and guilt-ridden over the nursing home placement decision. When the caregiver reaches her limit, she calls me for advice.

A rare dilemma for CPO policymakers is concurrent work by multiple physicians. Occasionally, two physicians legitimately share home care management. This is analogous to inpatient care, where several physicians are paid concurrently, and appropriately, for managing one seriously ill patient. Yet under CPO only one physician can be paid.

The requirement to document CPO work is a more substantive problem. Though it is not yet clear how much paperwork will ultimately be required by the many regional carriers who pay the bills for Medicare, physicians are advised to record all interactions. This is challenging. Sometimes phone calls from nurses come when physicians are away from the office. Even inside the office, documentation is difficult to create and collate. Many physicians feel that the hassle is not worth $60. Physicians are not used to counting and recording their work minute by minute, and 30 minutes of CPO can represent eight separate bits of work. I find that CPO documentation adds a meaningful, annoying burden but that adding 5 minutes of documentation to 30 minutes of unpaid care management is well worth $60. I have also experienced significant difficulties and payment delays with our regional carrier when billing for CPO.

WORK ISSUES IN THE CPO PROGRAM

In developing the CPO proposal the HCFA raised several issues, including potential cost and the need to clearly define the work involved. Chapter 2 gives more details on the latter.

The first work category involves medical decision making. Here are some sample questions from a 2-week period. Does the patient have a urinary tract infection or just bacteria in the urine? If it is an infection, what medicine should be used? A patient with heart failure has increased shortness of breath and asymmetric leg swelling; should we change the cardiac medications, or could this be a pulmonary embolus? A patient is taking Coumadin for a blood clot. Now the prothrombin time is markedly prolonged after being stable for 3 weeks, and there is blood in the stool. How should we adjust the Coumadin dose? What caused the change? And should we worry about the bleeding? Should the patient go to the emergency room? After giving telephone advice, I must later review and sign the related treatment plan revisions that come by mail.

A second category is caregiver support. Some caregivers need even more of the physician's time than patients do because they are unsure about the complex medical issues. They need a guide through the care process, asking many questions and sometimes simply needing to know that an ally is available.

A third category is monitoring quality and defining performance standards. Sometimes people fail to perform their job in a timely or effective manner. I spent 10 minutes on the phone because a lab service failed to draw the coagulation profile requested for an unstable anticoagulation patient and wanted to delay the repeat venipuncture for 3 days, creating the potential for serious complications.

A fourth category is oversight of home medical equipment and supplies. The new durable medical equipment regional carrier (DMERC) system is intended to remedy policy and procedure issues that have haunted home medical equipment certification. The DMERCs provide standard forms (CMNs) for various types of equipment, asking specific questions about the patients. This increases physician responsibility and may require chart review. If the work is done incorrectly, legitimate services may be denied, creating additional work to correct the problem. Home medical equipment certification is burdensome. At MCV Home Care, I receive as many as 10 CMNs per day, and I have rarely opened a day's mail that contained no CMNs or HME recertification orders.

Finally, when patients need specialized attention or acute care, the managing physician coordinates care with consultants or with providers in emergency rooms and hospitals. Home care physicians often are not compensated for coordinating care, whereas the acute care physicians and consultants are usually well paid for their work.

The HCFA asked about care management by professional providers, anticipating that physicians would request CPO payments for providers' work. My experience leads me to enthusiastically endorse such a team model. MCV Home Care nurse practitioners handle at least two-thirds of the care management. Each day, they direct the care of unstable patients. The question about treatment for a bladder infection would be routine for a nurse practitioner. The question about heart failure medications might also be handled if the nurse practitioner knew the case well. With problems like anticoagulation, the nurse practitioner might collect data, formulate a plan, and then ask physician advice because warfarin pharmacology is complex and the risk is high. Due to the medical complexity of our cases we must have good communication and active participation by physicians, even with experienced nurse practitioners. However, we are not paid for this work. This CPO policy should change.

The HCFA also expressed concern about beneficiary liability. Medicare patients are billed for co-payments from CPO charges, even though they may not have seen the physician for months. Those patients receiving home care have slightly more aggregate co-payments with CPO. However, Medicare physician payment is a closed system overall, so co-payments for all other services are fractionally less because of CPO. CPO co-payments are also small ($8), appropriate, and often covered by co-insurance. Moreover, Medicare home health care is heavily regulated, making it difficult for an unscrupulous physician to take advantage of Medicare beneficiaries under the CPO policy. HCFA further recognized that physicians are *required* to provide the care management service being compensated by CPO.

Most important, beneficiaries open to home health care now receive this physician service at no cost. Some of the work is direct contact with patients and families who call seeking advice. More is provided when physicians advise home health professionals. Patients are often unaware of the latter physician work, but this does not reduce its value.

Reviewing the first year (1995) of CPO payment teaches several lessons. First, only $45 million of approved charges were registered, compared with the $310 million Medicare anticipated. Speaking with physicians, it appears that hassles with documentation and lack of familiarity with the process were two important factors. Second, CPO billing was disproportionately higher in the South, to some extent reflecting regional variation in Medicare home health use. Finally, and most concerning, there are early reports of inappropriate physician use of the CPO code. This is currently under study.

THE FINANCIAL EFFECT OF HOME CARE ON PHYSICIAN OFFICE PRACTICE

Putting house calls and care management together, consider again the hypothetical office-based physician making a salary of $100,000, with gross income needs of $220,000. Assuming a typical 55-hour work week, 4 weeks of annual vacation, 20 homebound patients with active problems among 2,000 total patients, 10 1-hour house calls per homebound patient annually, and 3.5 hours per week in home care management, one finds home care consuming 15% of the physician's effort. If the home care load were 50 cases, they alone would require 35% of total effort. These concepts are shown graphically in Table 12.6, making no allowance for overhead reduction during house calls and using $83 per hour as an average total operating cost. The assumptions are obviously important. Delegating some house calls and care management to professional providers would free some physician time while increasing overhead; and simply providing fewer house calls altogether would lessen total cost, as would reducing office staffing during house call hours. In any case, the substantial nature of physician home care work must be well understood when designing equitable rewards under either fee-for-service or capitation payment.

GENERAL ISSUES IN COMPENSATION FOR HOME CARE PHYSICIANS

Care management is only one of several policy issues related to physician home care compensation. Another is the cost-effectiveness of house calls. This was addressed in chapters 9 and 10. It seems logical to value physician home care services no less than we value physician services for patients with chronic illness in other settings, such as the office or the nursing home. The work has many similar features, being primarily cognitive and being provided to patients with comparable clinical needs. Home care patients are if anything more challenging and more vulnerable and have less access to physicians than office or nursing home patients. As health care budgets tighten, closer scrutiny is being applied to high-volume, low-cost cognitive services, just as attention has already focused on utilization and efficiency of high-cost procedures.[21] Nonetheless, home care teams of physicians working with specifically trained professionals, whose training cost and salaries are lower, will undoubtedly gain importance.

Further formal study of physician home care work is urgently needed. The brief visit to check on a chronically ill patient, measure the blood pressure, and maintain continuity contrasts sharply with urgent home care or the ongoing management of medically unstable, seriously ill patients. All have value and should be encouraged when appropriate, but the time and difficulty vary, which should be reflected in the payment. There is a good foundation on which to build rational rewards for physician home care work that must now be refined. As president-elect of the American Academy of Home Care Physicians, I spent much time on this issue in 1995 and 1996. The process of changing the Medicare house call fee schedule has proved complex, convoluted, distorted, political, and slow.

TABLE 12.6 Weekly Cost of Home Care Work in Hypothetical Office Practice

| | Number of homebound patients | | |
Home care work	20	50	100
Care management	$332 (4 hr)	$ 833 (10 hr)	$1,660 (20 hr)
House calls 10 yr / patient 1 hr per house call	$346 (4.16 hr)	$ 865 (10.4 hr)	$1,729 (20.8 hr)
Total home care	$678	$1,658	$3,389
Percentage of gross income	15	37	74

POSSIBLE PROCEDURES FOR CHANGING HOME CARE COMPENSATION

Consider how physician home care compensation might evolve under two different overarching scenarios: fee-for-service payment and capitation payment. These create very different incentives. Under capitation, cost containment is the focus. Under fee-for-service, revenue generation dominates.

Some factors apply equally in both scenarios. For example, homebound patients always cause inefficiency in the office. Wheelchair or stretcher patients occupy extra waiting room space, require more nursing time for check-in, must be physically lifted on and off the exam table, require more nursing help for changing clothes and performing exams, and spend more time in the exam room. Seeing a severely impaired patient may take twice as long as seeing an ambulatory patient, sometimes with less information gained. Much of the work is done by office staff, but productivity is reduced and resources are consumed.

Another dimension where home care practice should be independent of the payment mechanism is care quality. I have argued that continuity of care, access to physician care, accuracy of patient assessment, reliability of postacute care follow-up with potential avoidance of unnecessary readmissions, and patient satisfaction are all improved by home health care and house calls. Regardless of the payment mechanism, one measure of success in a competitive health care marketplace will ultimately be a "report card" that includes quality measures. Strategic use of home care should improve the grade. Improved quality is an argument that helps me sustain hospital support for MCV Home Care.

Cost avoidance, another key argument for MCV Home Care, is a fiscal benefit realized under both payment mechanisms, but the effects differ, as discussed below. Likewise, the cost of providing most home care service is independent of the payment mechanism. Personnel, provider transport, "windshield time," record transcription, chart management, and billing costs are similar. The amount of care management work is the same in both payment models, as is office overhead, a continuing cost when office-based providers are outside the office. However, the impact of these costs may again differ with the payment mechanism.

THE FEE-FOR-SERVICE PAYMENT SCENARIO

"Loss-Leader" Concept

A feature of the fee-for-service scenario that has little relevance under capitation is the idea that reaching out to patients through house calls will secondarily benefit hospitals and specialists when the patients inevitably require acute care, consults, and procedures. Primary care physicians can also benefit secondarily through inpatient billing. More important for primary care, house calls help build practices. I have many office patients who are the relatives and neighbors of patients seen on house calls.

The loss-leader strategy works best where the penetration of managed care is low and hospitals are competing to fill beds with insured patients. Most homebound patients are insured by Medicare, Medicaid, or both. A much smaller percentage have private insurance as the primary payer. Under fee-for-service payment, hospitals and care systems should be inclined to support physicians and home care teams as loss leaders.

Cost Avoidance

Cost avoidance through home care is a two-edged sword under fee-for-service payment. Although the effect of home care on total health care costs remains uncertain, there is good evidence that home care shifts costs from acute care settings to the home. Hospitals are paid by the case under

Medicare DRGs. A shortened hospital stay means less inpatient resource consumption. Assuming that the DRG payment is unchanged, this should improve the hospital's bottom line. Also, some uncompensated "social" admissions for placement of patients in nursing homes can be averted or shortened by forward-thinking home care teams. This benefit may be partially offset if home care services attract new patients who are prone to long social hospitalizations.

In 8 years, 91 of 647 MCV Home Care patients (14%) entered nursing homes. Of these, 47 (51%) went directly to the nursing home, and 44 were hospitalized first. The mean duration of these hospitalizations was 32 days (range, 3–162). Most started with catastrophic illnesses that later forced institutional care, rather than being social admissions driven by caregiver burnout. A health care system with better integrated acute and long-term care would dramatically shorten some of the hospital stays that ended in nursing home transfers. Meanwhile, MCV Home Care patients had 990 other admissions, representing 9,332 bed days. We help our hospital financially.

On the other side of the ledger, experienced home care teams could actually reduce acute care revenues by solving problems at home that would previously have prompted emergency department and inpatient care. This effect is hard to measure. Generally, I believe that cost avoidance from shortened hospital stays outweighs "lost" revenues from preventing hospital care outright, because the illnesses that afflict homebound patients force facility-based acute care despite the best home care. Cost avoidance is a powerful incentive for hospitals to support interdisciplinary home care teams under present financing.

Under DRGs, hospital administrators thus consider these reasons for supporting medical home care: satisfying patient needs; providing a continuum of care with internal control over cost, quality, and access; reducing inpatient length of stay; and increasing new revenue.[22]

Financial Impact on Office Practice

As noted, the fee-for-service and capitation scenarios share the inefficiency that home care patients cause in the office, the disruptions caused by the acute problems of homebound patients and the burden of office overhead during house calls.

Care management is a different matter. Under fee-for-service payment, most care management work is "bundled" into fees for physician services in the office, hospital, or home. Here fee-for-service and capitation payment differ. In fee-for-service, to fairly compensate physicians for ongoing management of complex home care patients, there must either be a separate care management fee like Medicare's new CPO option, or direct encounter fees must be modified by patient-specific measures of complexity. These are hard to verify and document, and practical systems for measuring patient complexity are required. Capitation payers (see below) must still grapple with case-mix problems; however, capitation removes the pressure to generate the direct encounters that produce revenue under fee-for-service payment.

Other Concerns Under Fee-For-Service

A few physicians, faced with inadequate Medicare payments, have dropped Medicare participation and inform their patients that house call bills are the patient's responsibility. This is legal, but few elderly homebound patients can afford such bills. The same arguments apply to the practice of billing informed patients directly for home care services that are not covered by Medicare. If Medicare house call payments increased, such strategies would become unnecessary, and the increased co-payment burden would be modest.

Protection of Medicare beneficiaries from inappropriate house calls is another concern. When I started making house calls, I found that the first reactions of patients and families were gratitude and disbelief, but below the surface lurked concern about the cost. Most of my home care patients are relatively poor, and though I explain that I bill Medicare for house calls and accept assignment, some concerns persist. On the other hand, the Medicare Part B co-payment for a house call, now about $10, is tiny compared with the out-of-pocket cost from using ambulances, emergency rooms, and other means of accessing physician care.

Also, as previously mentioned, urgent home care is another quandary in the fee-for-service world. These problems disrupt other activities. Higher fee-for-service payments must be created for acute care house calls, reflecting the disruptive effects on other activities and the higher service intensity and prolonged service times.

Compensation of professional providers for home care work was also mentioned earlier. Because there is currently no Medicare reimbursement for house calls by professional providers, physicians with homebound patients in fee-for-service practices who consider sending associates on house calls have three undesirable options. First, they can accept this non-recoverable cost as being less expensive than the cost of diverting a more costly resource (the physician) from the office, and only partially offset by the house call payment. Alternatively, physicians could bill Medicare for a professional provider office service or a physician house call, risking charges of Medicare fraud. Finally, physicians could refuse to offer professional provider house calls.

We must also deal with perverse incentives. Fee-for-service payment encourages higher service volumes whenever a service is profitable, creating potential for abuse. The literature clearly documents wide, unexplained regional variations in the frequency of many procedures and costlier care when physicians own ancillary services. There is probably little current abuse of house calls, in part because the payment is so low. If and when house call payment exceeds the cost, the potential for overuse and abuse will rise, and monitoring utilization will be increasingly important.

Verifying physician work is another concern for regulators. In order of descending feasibility, verification is easiest in institutions like hospitals, nursing homes, or ambulatory care centers, less easy in ambulatory offices, and frankly difficult in home care. In home care there are few if any professionals who observe physicians at work, and many home care patients have limited ability to participate when investigating suspicious practices.

An administrator's nightmare might include an unscrupulous physician who visits adult homes or apartment buildings, sees many patients briefly and at more frequent intervals than is necessary and charges an inappropriately high intensity of service. The same skeptical administrator, previously burned, might picture physicians driving casually around town, intermingling personal errands and house calls, and billing for mileage and time as if the entire day were spent on home care. Although fraudulent, unethical, and far from the minds of most home care physicians, such possibilities must be considered. Unfortunately, a few physicians do abuse the system, and many more manipulate the system to maximum personal advantage.

Mechanisms for addressing these problems might include calculating a ratio of miles traveled per house call, adjusted for rural areas; tracking the number of annual home care services rendered to individual patients; and analyzing the number and intensity of home care services billed by a provider on a given day. Physicians whose practices appeared anomalous could be asked for more detailed information. These methods, however, are all somewhat cumbersome.

Another alternative would be to link physician home care payment to home health agency administration, where a detailed oversight process already exists. This might bring physicians and home health agencies together as a team, but it would also create serious problems. Many physicians work with multiple agencies, and agencies work with hundreds of physicians. The quality of communication between agency and physician varies and tends to be poor. Agency personnel would resent being burdened with physician oversight, and physicians might resent another bureaucratic intrusion. Further complicating matters, home health agency services are processed through Medicare Part A, whereas physician services use Medicare Part B. The regional administrators and databases are separate. Combined data from the two systems would be needed, and payment would be delayed. Also, Medicare home health agency care is intermittent, whereas physician care, at least theoretically, is continuous. Finally, linking physician payment to home health agency administration could create an undesirable conflict of interest between agencies and physicians. Thus, tying fee-for-service physician home care payment to home health agency administration seems inadvisable.

Then there is the full-time home care physician. For a few physicians, house calls are their principal clinical activity. Some, like MCV Home Care, are supported by systems of care, and a few exist independently. In a 1990 national survey of internists and family physicians,[3] one of 1,161 respondents reported 750 house calls per year, or 5 per workday, suggesting that home care was much of the practice. A second reported 400 house calls. Twenty-four physicians reported between 100 and 200 house calls each. There are now several organized home care practices, one involving over 20 physicians. Ancillary services like X ray, cardiac monitoring, and labs are an important part of their revenue stream.

I have many times considered a full-time home care practice. At a minimum, one needs a vehicle with a cellular phone and sophisticated information transmittal capability; portable medical equipment; an office with at least one staff member, where records are stored and phone calls are received and triaged; a billing service; access to advanced laboratory services; and malpractice coverage. The overhead for a mobile house call practice would be far less than the overhead for typical physician offices.

With lower overhead, full-time home care physicians might benefit unfairly from a house call fee schedule that factored in physician office practice overhead. Fee-for-service home care reimbursement might then be more equitable if home care physicians entered a registry, listing their practice setting and overhead burden, with an appropriate downward adjustment to home care fees.

THE CAPITATION PAYMENT SCENARIO

Loss Leaders

In this scenario, the first question of home care physicians is this: are you loss leaders or lightning rods? Under full capitation, including outpatient and inpatient care as in a Medicare HMO full-risk contract, the loss-leader concept has little value. Offering strong physician home care might provide transient advantages when competing to recruit enrollees. But homebound patients would be the last enrollees an HMO would want to attract, given the high prevalence of serious chronic illness and frequent need for expensive acute care. Rather, medical home care would be more quietly used to meet the needs of enrollees who developed complex problems while the marketing department targeted "healthy" individuals.

Cost Avoidance

This argument is strong in both fee-for-service and capitation scenarios and may be strongest under full capitation if the home care services are well managed. Not only would the capitated system seek to shorten hospital stays, but avoiding ambulance rides, emergency room visits, and hospital admissions would all be desirable. The biggest problem is the research, covered in chapter 6, which has not consistently shown system-wide cost savings after investing in home care. Home care costs rise when home care is encouraged. These added costs can overshadow savings from reduced inpatient and nursing home use unless home care is carefully targeted and well managed.

Abuse of the System

Physician abuse of home care is much less problematic under capitation. The beneficiaries have little financial risk, and managed care directors can monitor physician activity far more easily than can a centralized federal bureaucracy. The system manager's risk is that physicians might not be driven to work efficiently at home care. Home care has fewer tested mechanisms for monitoring work and measuring productivity.

Using Professional Providers for Home Care

This would be encouraged under capitation because current Medicare restrictions would no longer apply. Mature managed care systems with growing Medicare populations are developing interdisciplinary home care teams, including home care specialists, physicians who are responsible for delivering and managing home care for frail enrollees. These physicians may also have office or nursing home practices, but they are the capitated sector equivalent of full-time home care physicians in the fee-for-service sector.

Compensation

The biggest challenge for managed care systems is similar to the problem encountered under fee-for-service payment: how to value and compensate physicians fairly for the time they spend in home care.

One option is to screen enrollees, identify frail, potentially high-cost patients, separate them from the main capitation pool, and assign responsibility for directing and delivering their care to mobile physicians who are recognized and empowered as effective managers. This "carve-out" approach assumes that the physicians will continue to work hard and efficiently and deliver comprehensive care. Physician motivation can become problematic under capitation, resulting in reduced access, continuity, accountability, and comprehensiveness.[23] This can be addressed by estimating how many complex frail patients one physician or team can handle and then monitoring the census, services, outcomes, and patient satisfaction. Assigning frail patients to home care specialists also disrupts continuity of established physician relationships. This can be traumatic if physicians have remained actively involved in caring for their frailer patients. Still, I believe this option will ultimately prove most practical.

Another option is to adjust capitation rates by using measures of frailty, such as ADL impairments, or scores on predictive models. The need for case-mix adjustment is evident in one recent analysis that showed a 50% decrease in the coefficient of variation among HMO primary care physician practices after applying case-mix weights to outlier physician profiles.[24]

Using case-mix adjustment, one can increase reimbursement or, more likely, proportionately reduce physician panel size.

On a population-wide basis, such as the county-based system used in the Medicare AAPCC (adjusted average per capita cost), researchers have tried to adjust capitation rates by using chronic disease risk factors. This proved difficult.[25] Adjusting the AAPCC according to prior utilization of services also had limitations.[26]

On an individual patient basis, one might develop and apply a model such as the resource utilization groups (RUG) system, which has been shown to predict service use and cost in nursing homes.[27] Case-mix studies of episodes of home care have also shown potential, but problems remain.[28] Other recent work on alternative methods for paying home health agencies could eventually guide new physician home care payment models. In all, developing prospective payment for home care has been more difficult than similar efforts for nursing homes and hospitals, perhaps because unpredictable social variables have more influence on home care costs.[29,30] For example, a clinically sensible home care model with 18 patient categories explains only 10% of the cost variance; the 44-category RUG system explains 52%.[27]

Like a carve-out approach, the case-mix adjustment strategy entails separating high-risk patients from the larger pool by patient-specific individual measurements. Because capitation is normally calculated by using easily obtained demographic characteristics, like age or sex, that require no patient evaluation, case-mix adjustment would greatly increase administrative cost. Also, the patients tend to change rapidly, and keeping case-mix adjustments current is both difficult and expensive.

A third option is to use normal age and sex adjustments in capitation rates and let physicians take their chances. If a physician were unfortunate enough to attract disproportionately more complex frail patients, it would simply be tough luck. In primary care capitation for younger, employed populations, a panel of 1,000 patients is considered large enough to blunt the risk of adverse selection. However, when geriatric populations enroll in capitated care, the number of patients with complex care management needs rises exponentially, and the potential for physicians to become overextended or develop poor cost-effectiveness profiles increases sharply. This is particularly true for physicians who show interest or have experience in the difficult process of directing long-term care. Capitated physicians may seek to hide their geriatric skills.

Home Care Effects in Group Model
and Staff Model Arrangements

Home care effects may differ in group model and staff model capitation arrangements, and physician offices are potentially vulnerable to the differences. If staff model physicians are salaried, if their overhead is carried by the "system," or if they are designated as home care specialists, they are sheltered. However, consider a small independent physician office participating in a group-model HMO risk contract. If the practice acquired a disproportionate number of home care patients, it could create a serious problem unless the capitation schedule were very sophisticated or a special allocation was used to adjust for adverse experience. There exist precedents for fee-for-service payments to primary care physicians who receive capitation for most care, such as extra fees for annual women's health exams, peritoneocentesis, thoracentesis, or other time-consuming services.

GENERAL ECONOMIC CONSIDERATIONS

Much thought has recently been directed to the financing of long-term care, including home care.[31] Yet physician compensation for house calls and home care management has received little attention, partly because this has been a tiny fraction of physician services. In 1983, $98 *million* in charges (0.6% of approved Medicare physician charges) was recorded for physician house calls, compared with office charges of $4.7 *billion* and inpatient charges of $9.9 *billion*. Even in general practice and family practice, which have stronger home care traditions, physician house call charges were respectively only 2.6% and 2.0%. The number of house calls has remained low while home care has skyrocketed: in 1992 physicians authorized spending $12 billion for Medicare and Medicaid home health services, $5 billion for high-tech home care, and $13 billion for home medical equipment.

Thus, as home care expands and the physician's role inevitably and appropriately becomes larger and better defined, physician compensation for home care will need more attention. John Eisenberg, a noted scholar of health economics and physician reimbursement, articulately summarized the complex subject of physician motivation, practice pattern variations, and payment issues.[32] One key point was the importance of local culture and setting, being perhaps even more important than financial dri-ves. The example was the HMO, where the behavior of colleagues and the structure of the practice may be at least as important as perceived fis-cal effects from various activities. Six mechanisms for altering physician behavior were listed: education, feedback, participation, administrative changes, incentives, and penalties. Eisenberg felt that a combination would be needed, that no single avenue would suffice.

Victor Fuchs reminds us that health economics is inextricably linked with the larger socioeconomic context, using parents' unpaid medical min-istrations to their children, marketplace services like physician and hos-pital care, and public health issues like water fluoridation or automobile driving behavior as examples.[33] Home care is a subset of medical care that constantly verges on other societal domains, including caregiver avail-ability, housing, and transportation, all of which can dramatically affect the medical marketplace for home care. Fuchs notes that "every society needs an economic system because *resources* (natural, human and man-made) are scarce relative to human wants." We cannot afford unlimited health care, and we must make choices every day. A good economic sys-tem should offer: an optimum amount of resources devoted to health care; combination of resources in an optimal way, optimal distribution of health care, and optimal allocation of resources between current provision of care and investment for future health care (education, research, capital investment).

The U.S. economy is broadly characterized as a market economy. In the area of health care it diverges from the hypothetical perfect market that might be expected to produce optimum distribution of resources. Problems include paucity of sellers (e.g., hospitals); cooperation among sellers; restrictions on marketplace entry (licensing, certification, regula-tion); limited, unequal access to information that guides patient purchas-ing choices; and persistent disequilibrium between demand and supply. Specifically addressing physician payment, Fuchs notes that supply has been more important than demand in determining expenditures for physi-cian services.[33, chap 4] Interestingly, he uses house calls to exemplify a ser-vice for which demand exceeds supply and the going price is insufficient to bring supply and demand into balance, contrasted with surgical ser-vices, where supply exceeds demand.

A major feature distinguishing our system from a truly free health care market is inequality of access based on income, requiring compul-sory redistribution through taxes and insurance. Health care is therefore treated more as a right than a privilege. Fuchs criticizes undue fascination with technology as one cause of rising costs but says that this factor is not dominant. Ultimately, he believes that a better health care marketplace will be best achieved by encouraging individual responsibility and by controlling external social influences on health.

To forecast the future, Fuchs notes motivations in other sectors of our economy to control health care spending.[33, chap 17] Between 1950 and 1980, health insurance premiums increased from 6% to 40% of corporate profits and from 1% to 4% of disposable personal income. Federal health care spending rose from 4% to 12% of the federal budget, and health care increased from 4% to 9% of the gross national product. This led to major efforts at reducing hospital costs, the largest single component of health care expenditures. Fuchs identifies this as a critical aspect in the changing health economy. The shift to ambulatory care and home care is inevitable, as it is driven by powerful forces.

Fuchs concludes that the problem of health care financing cannot be completely resolved but that we can improve our approach by changing perceptions of what constitutes appropriate care. He cautions that preoccupation with cost containment creates the risk of providing inadequate coverage to many individuals, erosion of professional ethics, and loss of trust between patients and physicians. Ultimately, Fuchs believes that government must intervene on behalf of those less fortunate.

In closing this chapter, let me return to house calls as a small part of home care but an important marker of physician involvement and state that house calls are the experience on which other home care teamwork must be founded. It was through house calls that I came to truly understand home care, and it is house calls, sometimes quite infrequent, that make me a better home care team member. The results from the statewide mail survey of Virginia primary care physicians[4] and the national telephone survey of family physicians and internists[3] found remarkably similar numbers of physicians reporting that they would make more house calls if the reimbursement were increased. Nationally, 49% of physicians currently making house calls and 40% of those not making house calls indicated that they would increase house call efforts for greater reimbursement.

Though encouraging, this also suggests a need for a change in practice organization, because 53% of those making house calls and 80% of those not making house calls agreed that they were "too busy with office or hospital practice to make house calls." In addition, we must change medical education, training, and culture so that home care will expand sufficiently to meet the population's needs. Twenty-one percent of physicians who made house calls and 36% of those not making house calls disagreed with the statement: "I have sufficient knowledge about community resources to personally plan and deliver home health care." This brings us back to the picture of physician home care work as a mixture of direct care in the home and support for the interdisciplinary home care team. Both must be suitably recognized and encouraged.

REFERENCES

1. Public Policy Committee of the American Geriatrics Society. Home care and home care reimbursement. *J Am Geriatr Soc.* 1989; 37:1065–1066.
2. Adelman AM, Fredman L, Knight AL. House call practices: A comparison by specialty. *J Fam Practice.* 1994; 39(1):39–44.
3. Keenan JM, Boling PA, Schwartzberg JG, Olson L, Schneiderman M, McCaffrey DJ, Ripsin CM. A national survey of the home visiting practice and attitudes of family physicians and internists. *Arch Intern Med.* 1992; 152:2025–2032.
4. Boling PA, Retchin SM, Ellis J, Pancoast SA. Factors associated with the frequency of house calls by primary care physicians. *J Gen Intern Med.* 1991; 6:335–340.
5. Keenan JM, Bland CJ, Webster L, Myers S. The home care practice and attitudes of Minnesota family physicians. *J Am Geriatr Soc.* 1991; 39:1100–1104.
6. Boling PA, Keenan JM, Schwartzberg J, Retchin SM. Physician housecalls: Reimbursement is an issue. *J Am Geriatr Soc.* 1991; 39(8):A15.
7. Center for Health Policy Research of the American Medical Association. *Socioeconomic Characteristics of Medical Practice,* Chicago, Il: Author; 1993; p. 121.
8. Center for Health Policy Research of the American Medical Association. *Socioeconomic Characteristics of Medical Practice,* Chicago, Il: Author; 1991; p. 23.
9. Williams SJ. Ambulatory care: An overview and management introduction. Chapter 1, p 16. In: Ross A, Williams SJ, Schafer EL, eds., *Ambulatory Care Management.* Albany, NY: Delmar Publishers, Inc.; 1991.
10. Woodwell DA. Advance Data. National Center for Health Statistics. (No. 209). Washington, DC: Public Health Service, U.S. Department of Health and Human Services; 1992.
11. Gonzalez ML, ed. *Socioeconomic Characteristics of Medical Practice 1990/1991.* Chicago, Ill: Center for Health Policy Research, American Medical Association; 1991.
12. Master RJ, Feltin M, Jainchill J, Mark R, Kavesh WN, Rabkin MT, Turner

B, Bachrach S, Lennon S. A continuum of care for the inner city: Assessment of its benefits for Boston's elderly and high-risk populations. *N Engl J Med.* 1980; 302:1434–1440.

13. Zimmer JG, Groth-Juncker A. A time-motion study of patient care activities of a geriatric home care team. *Home Health Care Services Quarterly.* 1983; 4(1):67–78.

14. Hsiao WC, Braun P, Becker ER. Resource-based relative values. *JAMA.* 1988; 260:2347–2353.

15. Becker ER, Dunn D, Hsiao WC. Relative cost differences among physicians' specialty practices. *JAMA.* 1988; 260:2397–2402.

16. Hsiao WC, Braun P, Kelly NL, Becker ER. Results, potential effects, and implementation issues of the resource-based relative value scale. *JAMA.* 1988; 260:2429–2438.

17. Hsiao WC, Dunn DL, Verrilli DK. Assessing the implementation of physician payment reform. *N Engl J Med.* 1993; 328:928–933.

18. *Monitoring Access of Medicare Beneficiaries. Report of Physician Payment Review Commission to the U.S. Congress.* PPRC Report 94-2:8. Washington, DC, 1994.

19. *Federal Register.* 59(121):32765–32767. June 24, 1994.

20. Boling PA, Keenan JM, Schwartzberg JS, Retchin SM, Olson L, Schneiderman M. Reported home health agency referrals by internists and family physicians. *J Am Geriatr Soc.* 1992; 40:1241–1249.

21. Escarce JJ. Medicare patients' use of overpriced procedures before and after the Omnibus Budget Reconciliation Act of 1987. *Am J Public Health.* 1993; 83:349–355.

22. Lerman D. The hospital home care market. Chapter 1, pp. 1-16. In: Lerman D, Linne EB, eds., *Hospital Home Care: Strategic Management for Integrated Care Delivery.* Chicago: American Hospital Publishing, 1993.

23. Safran DG, Tarlov AR, Rogers WH. Primary care performance in fee-for-service and prepaid health care systems: Results from the Medical Outcomes Study. *JAMA.* 1994; 271:1579–1586.

24. Salem-Schatz SS, Moore G, Rucker M, Pearson SD. The case for case-mix adjustment in practice profiling: When good apples look bad. *JAMA.* 1994; 272:871–874.

25. Howland J, Stokes J, Crane SC, Belanger AJ. Adjusting capitation using chronic disease risk factors: A preliminary study. *Health Care Financing Review.* 1987; 9(2):15–23.

26. Beebe J, Lubitz J, Eggers P. Using prior utilization to determine payments for Medicare enrollees in health maintenance organizations. *Health Care Financing Review.* 1985; 6(3):27–38.

27. Fries BE, Schneider DP, Foley WJ, Gavazzi M, Burke R, Cornelius E. Refining a case-mix measure for nursing homes: Resource utilization groups (RUG-III). *Medical Care.* 1994; 32:668–685.

28. Branch LG, Goldberg HB, Cheh VA, Williams J. Medicare home health: A description of total episodes of care. *Health Care Financing Review.* 1993; 14(4):59–74.

29. Phillips BR, Brown RS, et al. Do preset per visit payment rates affect home health agency behavior? *Health Care Financing Review.* 1994; 16(1):91–108.

30. Goldberg HB, Schmitz RJ. Contemplating home health PPS: Current patterns of Medicare service use. *Health Care Financing Review.* 1994; 16(1):109–130.

31. Health and Public Policy Committee of the American College of Physicians. Financing long term care. *Ann Intern Med.* 1988; 108:279–288.

32. Eisenberg J. Physician utilization: The state of research about physicians' practice patterns. *Medical Care.* 1985; 23:461–483.

33. Fuchs VR. *The Health Economy.* Cambridge, Mass: Harvard University Press; 1986.

CHAPTER 13

Final Thoughts

I am a home care advocate, and I am sure that home care, applied correctly by a knowledgeable team, free of perverse incentives, located in a supportive system, and conscious of costs, is cost-effective. Setting aside the gratitude of patients and families, I have often seen medical, physician-led home care succeed wonderfully: clearly preventing hospitalization; clearly bringing patients into the hospital soon enough to have shorter, easier admissions for identical problems that a year before had caused much more complex admissions; clearly avoiding nursing home placement; and clearly helping patients recover who otherwise would have continued a life of greater functional limitation and discomfort. It pains me to read the many studies that have failed to demonstrate these benefits.

I am also a critic of home care. I have made house calls that could have been made by a nurse but that I was forced to make because federal policy did not allow ongoing nursing care to stable patients. I have seen home care resources wasted: excess services promoted, principally because of profit motives; patients and caregivers manipulating the system; inept providers derailing the process of care; and home care coordinated or delivered inefficiently. Thus, I can understand those who want to regulate or otherwise restrict home care and who have increased the attendant bureaucracy.

Some recent initiatives may yet succeed. One major barrier for community-based long-term care has been economic and bureaucratic compartmentalization of resources. Acute care is only loosely connected with skilled home care. Short-term home care and long-term home care run through different systems: Medicare and Medicaid. Nursing homes are often cut off from home care and acute care, and nursing homes may be inaccessible when there is an acute social need for alternative living arrangements, resulting in costly hospital care. Some patients have financial difficulty in obtaining basic home care, and the quality of those services is highly variable. In reporting that 35% or 40% of their work was done in the office, handling phone calls, paperwork, and other related tasks, the Rochester team echoes my own experience. Some of this effort is wasted yet is made necessary by an inefficient care delivery system. Approaches like PACE, social HMOs, and even managed care systems that arrange for contract nursing home beds, all seem to have organizational advantages.

The health care environment has also changed. Hospitalizations are dramatically shorter, and many serious problems are resolved outside hospital walls. Skilled home health care is more sophisticated. Some nursing home shortages have been rectified. Adult homes, board-and-care facilities, senior apartment buildings, and multilevel retirement communities are all more widely used. Communities, as the context of care, are evolving.[1]

Home care cost-effectiveness might be sensitive to the changing context, and medical home care may actually have greater impact. Although inpatient stays are shorter across all ages and diagnoses and ambulatory procedures are commonplace, homebound patients have illnesses that will require much inpatient care despite good outpatient services. As discretionary inpatient days are weeded out, homebound patients will consume a proportionately larger part of acute care. Programs that efficiently serve these patients would then have relatively more impact on overall acute care costs. Whether these programs can be *proved* to reduce overall system costs remains a question.

Another historical problem has been the small size of medical home care teams. A small team's efficiency is vulnerable to short-term staffing fluctuations, provider burnout or illness, and inability to use economies of scale for administration, purchasing, or coverage. In larger systems that include more individuals with home care expertise and capability, medical home care teams may function more efficiently. Nor has information technology been fully applied to medical home care, contrasted with hospital systems that use computers for on-line management of patient records. Better data management and new medical diagnostic and treatment technologies will soon enhance home care efficiency.

Finally, more research is needed. Experience tells me that there is value in continuous medical management, including physician involvement. The value is often hidden. It derives from awareness of patients' situations and baseline conditions, as well as from relationships established with patients and families, that later facilitate better decision making when inevitable health care or social crises arrive. Home care should be given because it is the best response to a legitimate need. Services should be targeted and customized to individuals' needs. Yet we must require efficacy, efficiency, and limitation of resources within constraints defined at a societal level.

Experimental home care trials are few in number, and they have been short. Weissert writes that these interventions have their greatest impact in a short period of time for any given case; with diminishing returns later. I believe that this relates in part to resource management. When the patient became permanently bedfast, did someone return the Hoyer lift to the medical equipment company, rather than continuing the rental? Did the medical team reduce its visits when patients stabilized? Did team members avoid excessive entanglement in untractable social conflicts?

I hope the future will see active exploration of the medical dimension in home care. Much of the work in long-term home care is socially driven and socially defined. Most of this work is done by unpaid caregivers. However, much of the budget for paid services involves medical dimensions, including acute care, a substantial part of institutional care, and some home care. Weissert writes:[1] "We provide nursing home care with little expectation of positive outcomes and complete certainty of increased expenditures. Since most who use home and community care are frail, dependent, sick, old, alone, or a burden to caregivers, why is it not enough to provide them with care which satisfies them? We expect even less of nursing homes."

Large-scale trials like PACE have the potential for broader generalizability and may help to foster a public policy that recognizes physicians as essential members of interdisciplinary community care teams. Most previous community-based care research has focused on the social dimension and neglected the medical dimension. New studies will also examine the situation-specific efficacy of medical home care interventions. In other cases, "social experiments" like the one now occurring with managed care, will develop solutions without the need for formal studies. We can profit from data gathered by managed care systems as they serve "difficult" populations by giving strategically defined resources to groups of selected, well-educated providers and letting them solve problems without first doing formal studies.

Returning together to earlier discussions of societal models, let's imagine the future. Assuming we are not devastated by nuclear holocaust, pollution, or a more natural disaster, I can see hazy outlines of a world where I may practice in 2020.

There will be more life care communities and extended multilevel facilities, housing a fraction of the elderly and of immobile younger people. Tastefully landscaped, user-friendly, and filled with relatively affluent residents, these places will be staffed with interdisciplinary medical teams and social support services. The teams will include physicians with a fairly comfortable role. Care will be coordinated and high in quality.

Urban apartment buildings designed to house and protect the vulnerable, the functionally impaired, and the less affluent frail elderly will be common. Again, care will be consolidated. Some buildings will have medical outreach clinics on-site; in others mobile provider teams will make rounds.

Nursing homes and adult homes will expand, for those whose needs exceed home care resources. Adult homes will offer more consistent quality, becoming low-cost nursing homes. Increasingly rare will be the physician with one or two patients per facility; increasingly common will be the long-term care specialist serving large numbers of patients in multiple settings.

Hospice care will grow, including options for terminally ill AIDS patients. However, the blurred margin between longer end-of-life home care and brief hospice care will remain, as people with chronic illness fight the approaching, yet indeterminate end.

The vast majority, the rest of the immobile population, young and old, will remain in the community, caught in the middle. Physicians and their teams will struggle with problems that are not easily solved. They will have a harder job than providers in settings where social issues are simpler. Systems of care and of payment for care will encompass many of these patients, but many more will remain near the cracks in the system.

The point where my crystal ball dims is the quality of home care we will provide. This will be a major moral test of our society. The technology to provide sophisticated, responsive, efficient home care exists. Will we develop a cohort of providers primed for home care and empower them to deliver it? Will we support informal caregivers or create economic pressures that force institutional care? How far will we extend home care to those who are only briefly ill or who want home care for convenience, using information technology instead of transportation?

Debates like the one over physician house calls will continue. Thirty years ago, skeptical, Fry challenged house calls' advocates to prove their worth.[2] Then, in "House Calls: Anachronism or Advent?" Goldsmith closed: "One could argue that either a large number of people are being denied an important service, or a small number are being given an inappropriate and inadequate one. Shouldn't we find out?"[3] Some such questions will be answered by research.

Regardless of which future emerges, we will certainly need to find more future physicians intrigued by home care and stimulate that nascent impulse. Some will choose to be "country doctors," like those in John McPhee's *Heirs of General Practice*. In this book about the careers of recent graduates from prestigious academic programs who chose rural primary care practice, he writes[4]:

> David Jones' farm consists of a house, a barn, a good-sized general-utility shed, and a hundred and four acres of land, some of which is wood-lot. An antique sign has been tacked up on an inside wall of the shed:
>
> LICENSED DOCTOR
>
> Healing
>
> Counseling
>
> House Calls Cheerfully Made
>
> The sign dates from the era of the horse-and-sleigh, but in each of its claims and proclamations it applies to David Jones. Cheerfully, he makes house calls—gets into his pickup, the back of which is full of farm hardware and pig feed, and, with his stethoscope on the seat beside him, goes to see a woman with severe back pain, an old man with shingles, a woman with cancer who is dying at home. These patients live in and near Washburn, Maine.

Some other emerging leaders in physician home care will find their niche in highly specialized clinical services, in administration, or in creating new technologies like the one, now available, that measures serum chemistries from a drop of blood. New home care leaders will pursue careers in health services research that will better inform us about home care, develop creative new financing alternatives, or work with those handling public money to make sure that it is spent but spent wisely.

Because I used much personal time to create this book, please permit me a final personal indulgence and a few reflections from my wilderness adventures. One of my pleasures is white water kayaking. I like to fight through boiling eddies, to follow the current when it is forceful but to guide my craft and gradually reach a goal, to work my way onto a glassy wave face and then glide motionless, the water slipping under my boat and the clean mountain air. There I can take pleasure in rewards from skilled effort and artistry and from my surroundings.

I clearly remember a few solitary minutes spent surfing on the face of a 15-foot wave at Serpentine Rapid in the heart of the Grand Canyon. I had paddled a quarter-mile back up the river to ride this huge wave. The sun was glistening through the spray from my paddle blades, and the water was icy cold and very fast at the bottom of the drop. Eventually, my arms grew tired, and a large raft appeared at the top of the rapid, so I slid off into an eddy. The guide waved and yelled, "Nice ride." Mine was a private epiphany, yet it is one I am glad to share.

The natural world is the place I go when I need to understand. There is something pure about mountaintops, broad oceans, open skies, wind, filtered sunlight or shade, gray days, storms, untamed rivers, fields, forests, and the creatures who inhabit these places. There is a natural order that puts the creative but often perverse and destructive human culture in perspective. When writing, I often find in myself connected to a pastoral movement, traceable back through the early American literary tradition. The same part of myself is attracted by the Navajo culture: belief in the power of the natural world to center human beings who are part of that world.

Then I return from the mountains, the rivers, or the mesas to the streets of Richmond, to the halls of our sometimes beleaguered public teaching hospital, to the homes of patients who are in pain or families who simply don't understand what to do about their situations. Renewed, it is easier for me to respond.

Providing home care is itself a small pastoral journey that can recall the others. Lest I be considered a hopeless romantic, be assured that I know well the dreary side of home care. Some house calls, like some trips in the mountains, are tedious, miserable affairs. However, others refresh me when I return to the hospital with its walls and its machines. I welcome other adventurers to join me in the brightening world of physician home care, and I salute my many partners in this endeavor.

REFERENCES

1. Weissert WG, Cready CM, Pawelak JE. The past and future of home and community-based long-term care. *Milbank Mem Fund Q.* 1988; 66:309–388.

2. Fry J. Home visiting: More or less? *J Fam Pract.* 1978; 7:385–386.

3. Goldsmith SB. House calls: Anachronism or advent? *Public Health Rep.* 1979; 94:299–304.

4. McPhee J. *Heirs of General Practice.* New York, NY: Noonday Press; 1984; pp. 17–18.

Index

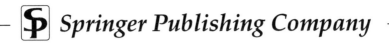
Home Care Nursing Services
International Lessons

Doris Modly, RN, MA, PhD, **Renzo Zanotti,** IP, AFD, PhD,
Piera Poletti, and **Joyce J. Fitzpatrick,** RN, PhD, FAAN

With home healthcare becoming a fast growing industry in the U.S., readers of this volume can pick up valuable lessons for their own institutions about how home health nursing is managed and structured in other countries around the world. Home health nursing experiences in ten countries are profiled, from Zimbabwe to Australia, along with overviews of important aspects of home health nursing world wide (such as education and research). Contributors include Ida Martinson, Violet Barkauskas, and Tina Marelli.

Contents:

1997   272pp   0-8261-9600-4   hardcover

536 Broadway, New York, NY 10012-3955 • (212) 431-4370 • Fax (212) 941-7842